O A R L

OXFORD AMERICAN RHEUMATOLOGY LIBRARY

Osteoporosis

O A R L
OXFORD AMERICAN RHEUMATOLOGY LIBRARY

Osteoporosis

Ronald C. Hamdy, MD, FRCP, FACP

Professor of Medicine
Cecile Cox Quillen Professor/Chair, Geriatric Medicine
Director, Osteoporosis Center
East Tennessee State University
Johnson City, TN

E. Michael Lewiecki, MD, FACP, FACE

Director, New Mexico Clinical Research & Osteoporosis Center
Clinical Assistant Professor of Medicine,
University of New Mexico School of Medicine
Albuquerque, NM

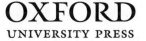

OXFORD
UNIVERSITY PRESS

OXFORD
UNIVERSITY PRESS

Oxford University Press is a department of the University of Oxford.
It furthers the University's objective of excellence in research, scholarship,
and education by publishing worldwide.

Oxford   New York
Auckland   Cape Town   Dar es Salaam   Hong Kong   Karachi
Kuala Lumpur   Madrid   Melbourne   Mexico City   Nairobi
New Delhi   Shanghai   Taipei   Toronto

With offices in
Argentina   Austria   Brazil   Chile   Czech Republic   France   Greece
Guatemala   Hungary   Italy   Japan   Poland   Portugal   Singapore
South Korea   Switzerland   Thailand   Turkey   Ukraine   Vietnam

Oxford is a registered trademark of Oxford University Press in the UK
and certain other countries.

Published in the United States of America by
Oxford University Press
198 Madison Avenue, New York, NY 10016

Library of Congress Cataloging-in-Publication Data

Hamdy, R. C. Osteoporosis / Ronald C. Hamdy, E. Michael Lewiecki.
p. ; cm. — (Oxford American rheumatology library)
Includes bibliographical references and index.
ISBN 978–0–19–992770–8 (pbk. : alk. paper)
I. Lewiecki, E. Michael.   II. Title. III. Series: Oxford American rheumatology library.
[DNLM: 1. Osteoporosis. WE 250]
616.7'16—dc23
2012029473

9 8 7 6 5 4 3 2
Printed in the United States of America
on acid-free paper

Dedication

We dedicate this handbook to our patients from whom we continue to learn so much.

Acknowledgments

Books do not generate spontaneously. We are deeply indebted to all our supporting staff for their patient help, particularly Jennifer Culp, Denelle Hensley, Lindy Russell, and Kathy Whalen. We are also grateful to the Oxford University Press staff, in particular Joan Bossert, as well as Aloysius Raj and his team at Newgen Knowledge Works for facilitating the project and keeping us on track. Last, but not least, we wish to thank our colleagues who refer patients to us, thus allowing us to gain a better understanding of managing patients with osteoporosis.

Disclosures

Ronald C. Hamdy's work as co-author of this book has been performed outside the scope of his employment as a US government employee. This work represents his personal and professional views and not necessarily those of the US government.

Other Support
  Amgen—speaker's bureau
  Novartis—speaker's bureau
  Eli Lily—speaker's bureau
  Warner Chilcott—speaker's bureau

E. Michael Lewiecki has received financial support or owned personal investments in the following categories during the past 1 year: Grant/Research Support (principal investigator, funding to New Mexico Clinical Research & Osteoporosis Center)
  Amgen
  Eli Lilly
  Merck
  GSK

Other Support
  Amgen—scientific advisory board, speakers' bureau
  Eli Lilly—scientific advisory board, speakers' bureau
  Novartis—speakers' bureau
  Merck—scientific advisory board
  GSK—consultant
  Warner Chilcott—speakers' bureau

Preface

"It was the best of times … It was the worst of times … It was the age of wisdom … It was the age of foolishness …" Charles Dickens' opening lines of *A Tale of Two Cities* accurately describe the present situation with osteoporosis.

We can easily diagnose osteoporosis. We know who and how to screen. Programs are available free of charge on the Web to estimate the individual patient's fracture risk and help clinicians focus on those at high risk, increasing the cost-effectiveness of the intervention and maximizing the risk:benefit ratio. Algorithms are available to facilitate and streamline clinicians' work. *Truly, this is the best of times … the age of wisdom.* And yet many patients are not diagnosed until a fracture occurs, and even after a fracture the diagnosis is often not made, increasing the risk of further fractures and increased mortality and morbidity. *Truly, this is the worst of times … the age of foolishness.*

We understand the role of various bone cells, how they interact with each other, and various factors affecting them. We develop medications that inhibit or activate these cells and design antibodies targeted at specific messengers to reduce bone resorption or increase formation. We have at our disposal medication to reduce the risk of fractures, even hip fractures. We know patients' fracture risk and the risk of various adverse effects. We can balance benefits versus risks of medications. Our efforts already have produced some encouraging results: The incidence of hip fractures is dropping in some countries. *Truly, this is the best of times … the age of wisdom.* And yet, many patients stop taking their medication and many clinicians are reluctant to prescribe medications for osteoporosis because of concerns about very rare possible adverse effects. *Truly, this is the worst of times … the age of foolishness.*

Osteoporosis is so common and its psycho-socio-economic impact so high that urgent action is needed, especially seeing that there are means to effectively reduce the risk of fractures before they occur. The numbers are such that the management of osteoporosis must be within the scope of primary care. Specialists have an important role, but most patients should be treated by clinicians providing primary care. This has been our main impetus while writing this book: to provide clinicians with an easily accessible, reliable, practical source of information—a handbook—to manage patients with osteoporosis. We have the means to change the natural course of osteoporosis, and reduce fractures and their dismal prognosis. We can do it, should do it, and must do it, but time is pressing.

RCH
EML

Contents

Chapter 1

Definition and Epidemiology

Osteoporosis is a disease characterized by compromised bone strength predisposing to an increased fracture risk.[1] It is asymptomatic until a fracture occurs. Although most fractures are acute dramatic events, many vertebral fractures are initially asymptomatic. Two main factors affect bone strength: bone mineral density (BMD) and bone quality (non-BMD determinants of bone strength). Whereas the former can be accurately and noninvasively measured by bone densitometry, bone quality as yet cannot be directly measured in clinical practice. Several intrinsic bone factors apart from BMD modulate the patient's fracture risk, including bone architecture, geometry, matrix properties, ratio of organic versus inorganic matrix components, collagen content, cross-linking, cement lines, degree of matrix mineralization, mineral crystal size, bone turnover, bone remodeling, and accumulation of microdamage (Fig. 1.1). Fracture risk is also increased by factors extrinsic to the affected bone, such as an increased propensity to fall.

OSTEOPOROSIS = INCREASED FRACTURE RISK

Bone Factors affecting fracture risk:
- BONE MASS/DENSITY
- BONE QUALITY

Figure 1.1 Bone Factors Affecting Fracture Risk.

Epidemiology

Osteoporosis is common and has significant psycho-socio-economic implications.[2] It is estimated that one in two women and one in five men over the age of 50 years old are at risk of sustaining osteoporotic fractures.[3] These fractures increase exponentially with age, and are often the result of trauma that ordinarily would not be expected to cause a fracture (fragility, low-trauma, low-energy, or low-impact fractures) or may occur spontaneously (atraumatic fractures). Although osteoporosis is a generalized disease and any bone may fracture, the most common sites are vertebrae, hips, distal radii, and proximal humerii.[4] Most osteoporotic fractures are preceded by falls.[4] A prior fracture increases the risk of future fractures (Fig. 1.2).

Hip Fractures

About 98% of hip fractures occur in patients over the age of 35 years, and their incidence increases exponentially with age. They are most common among

Incident Fracture	Hip	Vertebrae	Distal radius
Hip	2.3	2.5	
Vertebrae	2.3	4.4	1.4
Distal radius	1.9	1.7	3.3

Figure 1.2 Prior Fractures Increase the Risk of Future Fractures.
Adapted from Klotzbuecher CM, Ross PD, Landsman PB, et al. Patients with prior fractures have an increased risk of future fractures: a summary of the literature and statistical synthesis. J Bone Miner Res. 2000;15(4):721–39. Reprinted with permission from John Wiley & Sons, Inc.

white women; the female:male ratio is about 2:1. Most occur indoors and are the result of low trauma. A number of factors apart from osteoporosis and risk of falls may affect the fracture risk, such as hip axis length and femoral angle. This may explain discrepancies in fracture risk among different races and countries. In Europe, a threefold to 11-fold difference in the risk of fractures has been noted.[3]

Hip fractures are associated with a dismal prognosis: 24% to 30% excess mortality in the year following the fracture. About 50% of patients who were ambulant before sustaining the hip fracture are unable to walk independently after the fracture,[3] and about 20% require long-term nursing care.[5]

Vertebral Fractures

Vertebral fractures are the most common osteoporotic fractures and rarely result from direct trauma. Most occur while the patient is carrying on with daily activities.[4] Many are asymptomatic: only about one-third of patients with vertebral fractures have acute symptoms and seek medical help.[6] Most vertebral fractures are detected radiologically (morphologic vertebral fractures) when an x-ray is done for some unrelated condition. Regrettably, although this radiologic finding is noted in the radiologist's report, in many instances it is not included in the final summary, the vertebral fracture goes unreported, and no action is taken.[7] Consequences of vertebral fractures, even asymptomatic ones, include loss of height, back pain, kyphosis, protuberant abdomen, decreased lung vital capacity, loss of self-esteem, sleep disorders, depression, further fractures, and increased mortality. Once a fracture occurs, the risk of subsequent fractures is increased.[8]

Distal Forearm Fractures

Distal forearm fractures occur predominantly in women. Most are the result of a fall on the outstretched arm and are more likely to occur outdoors, especially in winter on icy pavements. Consequences of wrist fractures include pain, difficulties performing activities of daily living, degenerative arthritis, and reflex sympathetic dystrophy. More than one-half of patients who have sustained a wrist fracture report only fair to poor function 6 months after the fracture.[3]

Fractures of the Proximal Humerus

Fractures of the proximal humerus are usually associated with a fall to the side or obliquely forward, especially in patients who are not able to break their fall.[9] They are about three times more common in women than men. Main predictors include low femoral neck BMD, increasing age, loss of height, low daily calcium intake, and a propensity to fall.[10] Mortality is increased,[11] patients often require prolonged hospitalization periods,[12] and the ability to perform daily activities is often impaired.

Encouraging Trends

In the United States, the incidence of hip fractures has decreased from about 600 per 100,000 patient-years in 1997 to about 400 per 100,000 patient-years in 2007.[13] Similar findings have been reported in Canada, Australia, Switzerland, Finland, and other countries.[14–19] There is also evidence to suggest that the BMD of the femoral neck has increased in white women between the periods 1988–1994 and 2005–2008.[20] This may be the result of better patient and public health education, increased screening, and use of medications for osteoporosis.

References

1. NIH Consensus Development Panel on Osteoporosis Prevention, Diagnosis, and Therapy. Osteoporosis prevention, diagnosis, and therapy. JAMA. 2001:14;285(6):785–95.
2. Office of the Surgeon General (US). Bone Health and Osteoporosis: A Report of the Surgeon General. Rockville (MD): Office of the Surgeon General (US); 2004.
3. Harvey N, Dennison E, Cooper C. Epidemiology of osteoporotic fractures. In Rosen CJ ed. Primer on the Metabolic Bone Diseases and Disorders of Mineral Metabolism. 7th ed. ASBMR. Hoboken, NJ: John Wiley & Sons, Inc.; 2008:198–203.
4. Lauritzen JB. Osteoporotic fractures. In An YH ed. Orthopaedic Issues in Osteoporosis. CRC Press LLC.; 2003:171–73.
5. Chrischilles EA, Butler CD, Davis CS, et al. A model of lifetime osteoporosis impact. Arch Intern Med. 1991;151(10):2026–32.
6. Cooper C, Atkinson EJ, O'Fallon WM, et al. Incidence of clinically diagnosed vertebral fractures: a population-based study in Rochester, Minnesota, 1985–1989. J Bone Miner Res. 1992;7(2):221–27.
7. Gehlbach SH, Bigelow C, Heimisdottir M, et al. Recognition of vertebral fracture in a clinical setting. Osteoporos Int. 2000;11(7):577–82.
8. Klotzbuecher CM, Ross PD, Landsman PB, et al. Patients with prior fractures have an increased risk of future fractures: a summary of the literature and statistical synthesis. J Bone Miner Res. 2000;15(4):721–39.
9. Palvanen M, Kannus P, Parkkari J, et al. The injury mechanisms of osteoporotic upper extremity fractures among older adults: a controlled study

of 287 consecutive patients and their 108 controls. Osteoporos Int. 2000;11(10):822–31.

10. Nguyen TV, Center JR, Sambrook PN, et al. Risk factors for proximal humerus, forearm, and wrist fractures in elderly men and women: the Dubbo Osteoporosis Epidemiology Study. Am J Epidemiol. 2001;153(6):587–95.

11. Shortt NL, Robinson CM. Mortality after low-energy fractures in patients aged at least 45 years old. J Orthop Trauma. 2005;19(6):396–400.

12. Lübbeke A, Stern R, Grab B, et al. Upper extremity fractures in the elderly: consequences on utilization of rehabilitation care. Aging Clin Exp Res. 2005;17(4):276–80.

13. Nieves JW, Bilezikian JP, Lane JM, et al. Fragility fractures of the hip and femur: incidence and patient characteristics. Osteoporos Int. 2010;21(3):399–408.

14. Leslie WD, Sadatsafavi M, Lix LM, et al. Secular decreases in fracture rates 1986–2006 for Manitoba, Canada: a population-based analysis. Osteoporos Int. 2011;22(7):2137–43.

15. Lippuner K, Popp AW, Schwab P, et al. Fracture hospitalizations between years 2000 and 2007 in Switzerland: a trend analysis. Osteoporos Int. 2011;22(9):2487–97.

16. Chevalley T, Guilley E, Herrmann FR, et al. Incidence of hip fracture over a 10-year period (1991–2000): reversal of a secular trend. Bone. 2007;40(5):1284–89.

17. Kannus P, Niemi S, Parkkari J, et al. Nationwide decline in incidence of hip fracture. J Bone Miner Res. 2006;21(12):1836–38.

18. Fisher A, Martin J, Srikusalanukul W, et al. Bisphosphonate use and hip fracture epidemiology: ecologic proof from the contrary. Clin Interv Aging. 2010;5:355–62.

19. Pasco JA, Brennan SL, Henry MJ, et al. Changes in hip fracture rates in southeastern Australia spanning the period 1994–2007. J Bone Miner Res. 2011;26(7):1648–54.

20. Looker AC, Melton LJ 3rd, Borrud LG, et al. Changes in femur neck bone density in US adults between 1998–1994 and 2005–2008: demographic patterns and possible determinants. Osteoporos Int. 2012;23:771–80.

Chapter 2

Basic Bone Pathophysiology

Functions of the Skeleton

The skeleton is composed of bone and cartilage. It provides a mechanical structure for locomotion, support of soft tissue, attachment of muscles, and protection of vital organs. It encases bone marrow for hematopoiesis, immune functions, and hormonal activities. Bone is also a reservoir for calcium and phosphate to maintain mineral homeostasis.

Trabecular and Cortical Bone

There are two general types of bone: trabecular and cortical. Trabecular (cancellous) bone is the "sponge-like" bone found in vertebral bodies and near the ends of long bones. It comprises about 20% of total bone mass and 80% of bone surface area, with an annual turnover rate of about 25%. Cortical (compact) bone comprises the dense outer envelope of all bones. It makes up about 80% of total bone mass and 20% of bone surface area, with an annual turnover rate of approximately 3%. The macroscopic and physiologic differences between trabecular and cortical bone are clinically relevant with regard to rates of bone loss, fracture risk, and response to therapy.

In early postmenopausal estrogen-deficient women, predominantly trabecular bones such as the vertebrae have a higher rate of bone turnover, faster rate of bone loss, greater fracture risk, and faster response to pharmacologic therapy than bones that are mostly cortical, such as the mid-forearm. Because of its large surface area, high turnover rate, and close contact with soft tissues at endosteal surfaces, trabecular bone plays an important role in maintaining mineral homeostasis and extracellular acid-base balance. Cortical bone, with high density and ubiquity compared with trabecular bone, has important load-bearing functions.

Bone Mineral and Bone Matrix

Bone is a composite material consisting of organic and inorganic components. The organic matrix (osteoid) is about 98% type I collagen, with the remainder being a mix of non-collagenous proteins such as osteopontin and osteonectin. Type I collagen has a triple helix molecular structure with intramolecular and intermolecular crosslinks, providing scaffolding for the deposition of bone mineral. The inorganic mineral component of bone, which makes up about 70% of bone weight, is mainly calcium phosphate deposited as platelike nanocrystals in the gaps of collagen fibrils.[1] Other components of the mineral content include carbonate, magnesium, and fluoride. The composite nature of bone is analogous to reinforced concrete, with the collagen (like rebar) providing resistance to bending, and the mineral (like concrete) providing resistance to compressive loads. Disruptions in the quality, quantity, or balance of these components can reduce bone strength and increase fracture risk.

Bone Remodeling

Bone remodeling (turnover) is the dynamic process by which bone is continually removed and replaced in discrete locations called bone multicellular units (BMUs). There are approximately 1 million functioning BMUs in a healthy adult skeleton at any one time, replacing 8% to 10% of bone mass each year. On the surface of trabecular bone, a BMU takes the form of a cavity or trench (a hemi-osteon), whereas in cortical bone it is a tunnel-like structure called an osteon. In healthy young adults, the bone remodeling rate is generally low, with bone resorption approximately equal to bone formation. This results in a steady state of bone mass and good bone strength (Fig. 2.1).

In estrogen-deficient postmenopausal women, the rate of bone remodeling is accelerated and bone resorption exceeds bone formation. The driving force is an increase in receptor activator of nuclear factor kappa-B ligand (RANKL) caused by decreased estrogen production, resulting in a high rate of bone resorption (discussed later in this chapter). Bone strength is diminished because of several factors, including degradation of bone microarchitecture (e.g., trabecular thinning, trabecular perforation, loss of trabecular connectivity, cortical porosity, and cortical thinning), high number and large volume of BMUs resulting from a high rate of bone turnover, and net loss of bone that occurs when resorption exceeds formation.

The rate of bone loss begins to accelerate during menopausal transition, 2 to 3 years before the last menses, and continues for about 3 to 4 years after menopause. On average, women may lose about 2% of bone annually during this time, followed by a slower age-related bone loss rate of 1% to 1.5% per year.[2] The rate of bone loss varies according to skeletal site, generally being greatest at the lumbar spine, which has a high content of trabecular bone, and lower at the femoral neck, which contains a higher proportion of cortical bone. As a consequence of high bone turnover, the BMUs are larger and more numerous. Each of these represents a weakened area of bone (stress riser) that may be a

	Bone Turnover	**Bone Mass**
Children, Adolescents	Formation > Resorption	Increases
Adults	Formation = Resorption	Unchanged
Postmenopausal, Older Adults	Formation < Resorption	Decreases

Figure 2.1 Bone Is an Active, Dynamic Tissue.

focal point for the development of microcracks. An excess of BMUs leads to thinning of the trabeculae and increased porosity of cortical bone. High bone turnover is a risk factor for fracture independent of BMD.[3,4]

There are five sequential stages of bone remodeling—activation, resorption, reversal, formation, and termination. Activation of a BMU occurs when "resting" bone covered by lining cells is disrupted by mechanical strain, resulting in structural damage to bone (targeted remodeling) or by signaling associated with regulation of mineral homeostasis (nontargeted remodeling). Resorption begins when preosteoclasts are recruited to become well-differentiated mature osteoclasts that attach to the bone surface. Following bone resorption, there is a brief reversal phase, and then osteoblastic bone formation with deposition of osteoid that becomes mineralized. Finally, there is a termination phase in which some osteoblasts become osteocytes that are encased within the bone, and the bone surface is restored to its "resting" state covered by lining cells (also former osteoblasts) until the next bone remodeling cycle begins (Fig. 2.2).

All medications currently used for the treatment of postmenopausal osteoporosis affect bone remodeling.[5] Antiresorptive drugs primarily reduce bone resorption, whereas osteoanabolic drugs primarily increase bone formation. Antiresorptive agents strengthen bone and reduce fracture risk by decreasing bone turnover. This reduces the bone remodeling space and stabilizes or increases BMD through prolongation of secondary mineralization, with preservation of bone microarchitecture, reduction in trabecular perforation, and

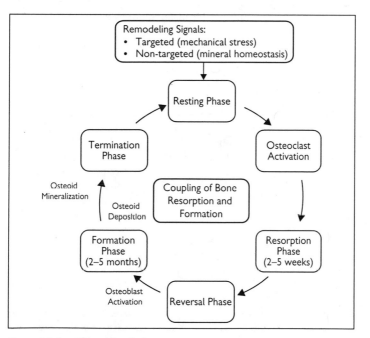

Figure 2.2 Bone Remodeling Cycle.

decrease in cortical porosity. However, lost bone is not replaced, and degraded bone microarchitectural elements are not restored. Osteoanabolic drugs strengthen bone and reduce fracture risk by increasing bone formation. They are associated with an increase in cortical thickness and restoration or formation of new trabecular microarchitectural elements.

Bone Cells: Osteoclasts, Osteoblasts, and Osteocytes

Bone remodeling requires the coordinated activity of three types of cells—osteoclasts (bone resorbing cells), osteoblasts (bone forming cells), and osteocytes (cells that detect mechanical loads applied to bone). This is normally a "coupled" process because of communication among these cells, whereby changes in bone resorption and formation are typically in the same direction (i.e., increased or decreased), although the magnitude of these changes may differ. Some drugs or combinations of drugs may "uncouple" bone resorption and formation, leading to opportunities for enhanced therapeutic effect.[6] The initiation of bone remodeling may be targeted to a specific location, such as the site of bone microdamage caused by mechanical loading, or untargeted in response to metabolic demands to maintain mineral homeostasis.[7]

Osteoclasts

Osteoclasts are large multinucleated cells originating from hematopoietic stem cells. The final common pathway for regulation of osteoclast differentiation, activity, and survival is RANKL, a cytokine expressed by osteoblasts and other cells. When RANKL activates its receptor (RANK) on the cell surface of preosteoclasts and mature osteoclasts, there is an increase in osteoclast formation, activity, and survival. Osteoprotegerin (OPG) is a soluble decoy receptor also produced by osteoblasts that serves a counter-regulatory function by binding to RANKL and preventing it from activating RANK. The balance between RANKL and OPG is a major determinant of the rate of bone resorption. Osteoblast expression of RANKL and OPG is controlled by many growth factors, hormones, cytokines, and drugs (Fig. 2.3).

The attachment of the osteoclast to the bone surface occurs by means of a "sealing zone," creating a self-contained area between ruffled border of the osteoclast and bone surface. Here, enzymes such as cathepsin K degrade the protein matrix, whereas the acidic microenvironment dissolves the bone mineral. Terminal peptide fragments of type I collagen, such as N-telopeptide (NTX) and C-telopeptide (CTX), pyridinium crosslinks, deoxypyridinoline, and pyridinoline are examples of bone resorption markers. These are released into the circulation and can be measured in the serum and/or urine, providing an indirect assessment of the rate of bone resorption.

Other compounds derived from the bone matrix or produced by osteoclasts may communicate with osteoblasts to regulate the next phase of remodeling. Osteoclastic bone resorption typically occurs over 2 to 5 weeks and ends with apoptosis, or programmed cell death, of osteoclasts. During a transitory reversal phase that immediately follows bone resorption, collagen remnants

Cell Type	Function(s)	Principal Regulator(s)	Markers of Activity	Fate
Osteoclasts	Bone resorption	RANKL, Cathepsin-K	NTX, CTX, Pyridinium crosslinks	Apoptosis
Osteoblasts	Bone formation	Ephrin	Osteocalcin	Osteocytes
	Express RANK-L & OPG	Wnt-β-catenin	Bone-specific alkaline phosphatase	Lining cells
	Activate osteoclasts	TGF-β, IGF-1	Procollagen molecules P1NP & P1CP	Apoptosis
Osteocytes	Mechano-sensing	Mechanical stress		Apoptosis
		Sclerostin (inhibits Wnt-β-catenin)		

Figure 2.3 Major Bone Cell Types, Functions, Regulators, and Markers of Activity.

are removed and the bone surface is prepared for bone formation. The cells responsible for the reversal phase are poorly characterized, but appear to be mononuclear cells that may include monocytes, former osteocytes, and preosteoclasts.

Osteoblasts

Osteoblasts are bone-forming cells derived from mesenchymal stem cells. They produce the protein bone matrix, primarily type I collagen, that partially or completely fills the cavity produced by osteoclasts and subsequently becomes mineralized. Ephrin signaling may play a role in the initiation of osteoblast differentiation during the reversal phase through close interplay among osteocytes, osteoclasts, and osteoblasts.[8] Osteoblast differentiation is activated through the canonical Wnt/β-catenin pathway by Wnt signaling proteins that bind to a transmembrane coreceptor on the osteoblast cell surface. Osteoclast-derived signaling molecules such as transforming growth factor β (TGF-β) and insulin-like growth factor 1 are released during bone resorption and appear to regulate the activity of mature osteoblasts.

The process of bone formation occurs over 2 to 5 months. Active osteoblasts secrete compounds including osteocalcin, bone-specific alkaline phosphatase, and procollagen molecules that undergo enzymatic cleavage-yielding terminal peptide fragments, procollagen type I N-propeptide (P1NP) and procollagen type I C-propeptide (P1CP). These markers of bone formation are released into the circulation and can be measured in the serum, providing an indirect assessment of the rate of bone formation. Primary mineralization of newly formed osteoid occurs rapidly, with about 70% of mineralization completed within several days, whereas the long-term process of secondary mineralization proceeds over months to years. The fate of osteoblasts on completion of the bone formation phase is to disappear by apoptosis, become lining cells on the bone surface, or osteocytes encased in bone.

Osteocytes

Osteocytes, by far the most numerous and long-lived bone cells, are found in lacunae throughout the bone matrix. They communicate with one another and with bone lining cells through a network of cytoplasmic connections within bone canaliculi.[9] Osteocytes express sclerostin, a molecule that inhibits Wnt signaling and reduces osteoblastic bone formation, as well as TGF-β, a molecule that inhibits osteoclastogenesis and/or osteoclast activity. Osteocytes act as mechanosensors that can detect load or stress applied to bone and play an important role in orchestrating targeted bone remodeling. Osteocytes appear to respond to mechanical stress by undergoing apoptosis, which in turn leads to osteoclastogenesis.[8]

Bone Turnover Markers

Bone turnover markers (BTMs) are biochemical byproducts of bone resorption and formation that can be measured in the blood and/or urine with commercially available laboratory assays. Postmenopausal women with elevated BTM levels have reduced BMD,[4] higher rates of bone loss,[10] and increased fracture risks[11] compared with women with lower BTM levels.

The clinical use of BTM requires a thorough understanding of their limitations. Numerous sources of variability confound the interpretation of BTM levels. Uncontrollable sources of variability include age, sex, menopausal status, fractures, pregnancy, lactation, comorbidities, drugs, and immobility.[12] Controllable sources of variability include time of day, fasting status, and exercise.[12] There is also analytical variability associated with methods of processing the specimen and assay used. BTM reference ranges vary according to the type of BTM and reference population.

Calcium Metabolism

The skeleton is a readily available source of calcium. Adequate intracellular, extracellular, and serum calcium levels are essential for most cellular activities, and several homeostatic mechanisms interact to maintain the serum calcium level within a narrow range of normality. Calcium homeostasis takes precedence over mechanical integrity of the skeleton.

Whenever the serum calcium level decreases, it stimulates the release of parathyroid hormone (PTH), which stimulates the osteoclasts to increase bone resorption and mobilization of calcium from skeleton to circulation. PTH also increases renal tubular calcium resorption. In the kidneys, PTH stimulates 1-alpha-hydroxylase enzyme to hydroxylate 25-hydroxyvitamin D to 1,25 di-hydroxyvitamin D—the most active vitamin D metabolite—which increases the active absorption of calcium through the gastrointestinal tract (Fig. 2.4).

When the serum calcium level increases, less PTH is released, osteoclastic activity is reduced, less calcium is mobilized from bones to circulation, less calcium is reabsorbed by the renal tubules, and the hydroxylation of 25-hydroxyvitamin D yields metabolically inactive metabolites that do not increase

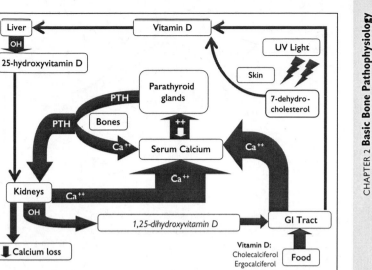

Figure 2.4 Hypocalcemia-Triggered Homeostatic Mechanisms.

the intestinal absorption of calcium. If—despite all these compensatory mechanisms—the serum calcium level increases, it stimulates the production of calcitonin from the C-cells of the thyroid gland. Calcitonin reduces bone resorption by inhibiting the osteoclasts and increases the renal tubular calcium excretion. Salmon calcitonin is the most potent calcitonin, probably because during its migratory journey salmon moves rapidly from a low calcium environment (fresh water) to a high calcium environment (sea water) and has to rapidly increase renal calcium excretion to avoid hypercalcemia (Fig. 2.5).

Vitamin D Metabolism

Vitamin D can be formed in the skin by the action of ultraviolet light on 7-dehydro-cholesterol, converting it to cholecalciferol. Alternatively, vitamin D may be obtained from ingested animal food (cholecalciferol), or ingested plants (ergocalciferol). Both follow the same metabolic pathway, hydroxylated at the 25-position to form 25-hydroxyvitamin D in several organs, but predominantly in the liver. Both are then hydroxylated in the kidneys, either at the 1-position to yield 1,25-di-hydroxy-vitamin D, or at other positions to yield inactive metabolites. Available bioassays can differentiate the various metabolites.

Vitamin D deficiency and insufficiency are common even in sunny temperate areas.[13] There are no specific clinical features. Patients with very low vitamin D levels may experience generalized aches and pains, bone tenderness, proximal myopathy, and a waddling gait. Nonspecific neuropsychiatric symptoms are sometimes seen, including fatigue, lethargy, and depression. The diagnosis is established by assaying the serum 25-hydroxy-vitamin D level. The serum

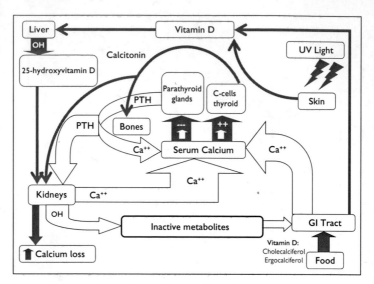

Figure 2.5 Hypercalcemia-Triggered Homeostatic Mechanisms.

PTH level may be elevated as a compensatory mechanism to compensate for the negative calcium balance; serum 1,25-di-hydroxy-vitamin D may be normal in response to elevated PTH levels. Urinary calcium excretion is reduced. The serum calcium level remains within normal range until calcium homeostasis is no longer able to compensate. The serum alkaline phosphatase may be marginally elevated.

In patients with renal impairment, the assay of 1,25-di-hydroxy-vitamin D is useful because it indicates whether or not the kidneys are able to hydroxylate 25-hydroxy-vitamin D at the one-position to produce the active vitamin D metabolite. This has therapeutic implications in choosing the vitamin D supplement. Patients who cannot hydroxylate 25-hydroxy-vitamin D will not increase 1,25-di-hydroxy-vitamin D levels with the administration of cholecalciferol or ergocalciferol and should be prescribed active vitamin D metabolites such as 1,25-di-hydroxy-vitamin D. In that instance, however, the serum calcium level should be carefully monitored, as the body's homeostatic mechanisms are bypassed and hypercalcemia may occur.

There is no consensus on optimum vitamin D supplementation in patients with hypovitaminosis D. Regimens include ergocalciferol 50,000 units once a week or cholecalciferol 2,000 to 5,000 units daily for 8 to 12 weeks. Re-assaying serum 25-hydroxy-vitamin D is recommended at the end of the course. There is also no consensus regarding the optimum maintenance doses once the serum vitamin D level has normalized; the US National Osteoporosis Foundation suggests vitamin D 800–1000 IU per day for postmenopausal women and men age 50 years and older, with titration of the dose to maintain a desirable blood level. A repeat assay of the serum vitamin D level annually, preferably at the end of the winter period when the body's stores are at their lowest level, is sometimes recommended to ensure the patient does not relapse into hypovitaminosis D.

References

1. Robey PG, Boskey AL. The composition of bone. In Rosen CJ ed. Primer on the Metabolic Bone Diseases and Disorders of Mineral Metabolism. ASBMR. Hoboken, NJ: John Wiley & Sons, Inc.; 2008:32–38.

2. North American Menopause Society. Management of osteoporosis in postmenopausal women: 2010 position statement of The North American Menopause Society. Menopause. 2010;17(1):25–54.

3. Garnero P, Hausherr E, Chapuy MC, et al. Markers of bone resorption predict hip fracture in elderly women: the EPIDOS Prospective Study. J Bone Miner Res. 1996;11(10):1531–38.

4. Garnero P, Sornay-Rendu E, Chapuy MC, et al. Increased bone turnover in late postmenopausal women is a major determinant of osteoporosis. J Bone Miner Res. 1996;11(3):337–49.

5. Riggs BL, Khosla S, Melton LJ III. The assembly of the adult skeleton during growth and maturation: implications for senile osteoporosis. J Clin Invest. 1999;104(6):671–72.

6. Lewiecki EM. Combination therapy: the Holy Grail for the treatment of postmenopausal osteoporosis? Curr Med Res Opin. 2011;27(7):1493–97.

7. Burr DB. Targeted and nontargeted remodeling. Bone. 2002;30(1):2–4.

8. Henriksen K, Neutzsky-Wulff AV, Bonewald LF, et al. Local communication on and within bone controls bone remodeling. Bone. 2009;44(6):1026–33.

9. Bonewald LF. Osteocytes. In Rosen CJ ed. Primer on the metabolic bone diseases and disorders of mineral metabolism. ASBMR. Hoboken, NJ: John Wiley & Sons, Inc.; 2008:22–27.

10. Ross PD, Knowlton W. Rapid bone loss is associated with increased levels of biochemical markers. J Bone Miner Res. 1998;13:297–302.

11. Gerdhem P, Ivaska KK, Alatalo SL, et al. Biochemical markers of bone metabolism and prediction of fracture in elderly women. J Bone Miner Res. 2004;19:386–93.

12. Hannon R, Eastell R. Preanalytical variability of biochemical markers of bone turnover. Osteoporos Int. 2000;11 Suppl 6:S30–44.

13. Hollick MF. Vitamin D deficiency. N Engl J Med. 2007;357:266–81.

Chapter 3

Bone Densitometry and Other Technologies

Bone density is the single most important factor affecting bone strength. Bone densitometry is a noninvasive bone imaging technique to assess the density of select bones.

Dual-Energy X-Ray Absorptiometry

Targeted bones are exposed to a known quantity of energy. The amount of energy absorbed by the bones reflects their mineral content. Two separate waves of energy—absorbed to different degrees by soft and bone tissue—are used to differentiate bone from soft tissue, hence the name dual-energy x-ray absorptiometry (DXA).

The only two direct measurements made during bone densitometry are bone mineral content (BMC, in grams [g]) and surface area (cm²) of the bone scanned. The former is then divided by the latter to calculate bone mineral density (BMD, in g/cm²). The patient's BMD is then compared with that of a young-adult sex-matched reference population to calculate a T-score, and an age-, sex-, and ethnicity-matched population to calculate a Z-score. The T-score and Z-score are the number of standard deviations the patient's BMD differs from the mean BMD of the young-adult and age-matched populations, respectively (Fig. 3.1).

Different Densitometers Use Different Technologies

The manufacturers of bone densitometers use different technologies to produce the two waves of energy and different algorithms to differentiate bone tissue from soft tissue. As a result, the absolute values of BMD, BMC, and surface area of bone scanned are not the same with all densitometers. Furthermore, manufacturers designate different areas of the anatomic femoral neck as the *femoral neck*. For example, GE Lunar designates this area as the mid-point of the hip axis, whereas Hologic designates it as the area immediately adjacent to

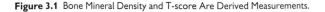

$$BMD = \frac{Bone\ Mineral\ Content}{Surface\ area\ of\ bone\ scanned}$$

$$T\text{-score} = \frac{Patient's\ BMD - Reference\ Population\ Mean\ BMD}{Standard\ Deviation\ of\ Reference\ Population}$$

Figure 3.1 Bone Mineral Density and T-score Are Derived Measurements.

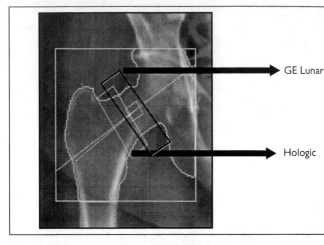

Figure 3.2 "Femoral Neck" Is Anatomically Different in GE Lunar and Hologic DXAs.

the greater trochanter (Fig. 3.2). Therefore, it is not possible to use absolute BMD values for diagnostic purposes; hence, the use of T-scores.

Factors Affecting Accuracy of Dual-energy X-ray Absorptiometry

Bone densitometry is a well-established tool for measurement of BMD. Great strides have been made to ensure maximum accuracy and reproducibility. Like most tools, however, the results are also dependent on the skills of the technologist performing the scans. Several factors extraneous to the densitometer may affect the scan results, including the following.

Ability of the Technologist to Position the Patient Correctly on the Scanner Table

Relatively small changes in the patient's position may result in differences in BMC, bone area, and consequently, BMD and T-scores. If the patient's leg is too abducted or adducted, or if it is not sufficiently rotated, the bones will be scanned from different angles and different results may be obtained because the bone cross-sections are not cylindrical, but oblong. For this purpose, strict criteria have been proposed by the International Society for Clinical Densitometry (ISCD) to ensure the quality of the scans and their usefulness to diagnose the patient's bone status and monitor progress.

The ISCD also recommends that precision assessment be routinely done to calculate the least significant change (LSC) for each technologist where the DXA scans are done.[1] Precision assessment with phantoms is not the same as with patients, as the repositioning of a phantom does not involve the same problems as repositioning patients. Without knowing the LSC, it is not possible to determine the statistical significance of an observed change over a period of time (see Chapter 9). Calculating the precision and LSC is not considered research, but quality assurance.[2] Detailed methodology on how to calculate precision is available on the ISCD web site www.iscd.org.

Given the importance of patient positioning, it is valuable for clinicians to review the scan images to assure that positioning is correct and that serial studies are comparing skeletal sites that are positioned in the same way.

Characteristics of a Well-positioned Proximal Femur Scan (Fig. 3.3)

1. The proximal femur is surrounded by soft tissue.
2. There are no artifacts.
3. The femoral shaft is perpendicular, neither abducted nor adducted.
4. The lesser trochanter is barely visible to ensure the degree of leg rotation is adequate.
5. The femoral neck box:
   a. Is adequately placed: anchored to the greater trochanter for Hologic scanners and mid-point of the hip axis for GE Lunar.
   b. Contains only the femoral neck. If the ischium is too close to the femoral neck, a software application is available to exclude it from the analysis.

Following are some common examples of improper techniques (Figs. 3.4–3.6). Sometimes this is unavoidable if the patient has an arthropathy or is in pain. The technologist should include this observation in the report and ensure that the patient is placed in exactly the same position in follow-up scans.

Characteristics of a Well-positioned Lumbar Spine Scan

1. The vertebrae are located in the center of the image, with an equal amount of soft tissue on either side.
2. The lower ribs are visible.
3. The iliac crest is visible.
4. There are no artifacts.
5. The lines on the intervertebral discs are properly placed and correctly labeled (Fig. 3.7).

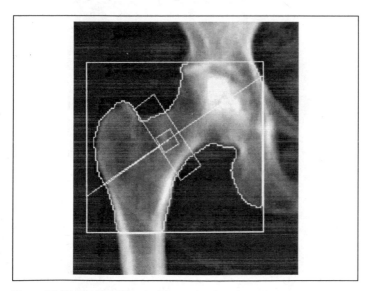

Figure 3.3 Well-Positioned Proximal Femur.

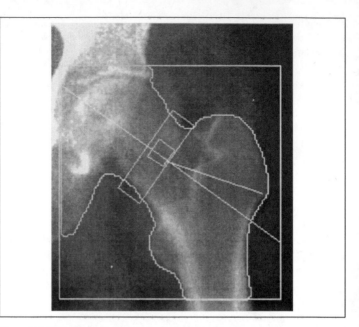

Figure 3.4 Lesser Trochanter too Prominent.

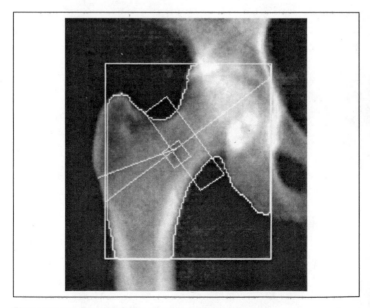

Figure 3.5 Not Enough Soft Tissue Lateral Aspect of Femur.

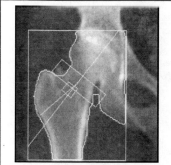

| Femoral neck box includes pelvic bone, software available to exclude pelvic bone | Pelvic bone excluded from analysis using software |

Figure 3.6 The Femoral Neck Box Should Only Include the Femoral Neck.

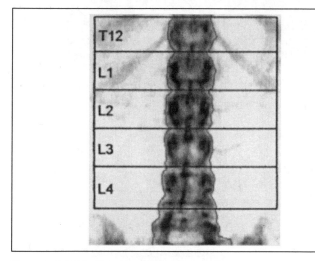

T12
L1
L2
L3
L4

Figure 3.7 Well-Positioned Lumbar Vertebrae.

Characteristics of a Well-positioned Distal Radius and Ulna Scan

1. The bones are parallel and centered.
2. One row of carpal bones is visible.
3. There are no artifacts.
4. Dense cortical bone in distal radius is excluded from the region of interest (Fig. 3.8).

The Presence of Artifacts in the Path of the Energy Waves

These artifacts could be within the patient's body, such as osteophytes, scoliosis, and orthopedic hardware, or extraneous to the patient, such as metal buttons, zippers, naval rings, and decorative accents on clothing or a wallet inadvertently

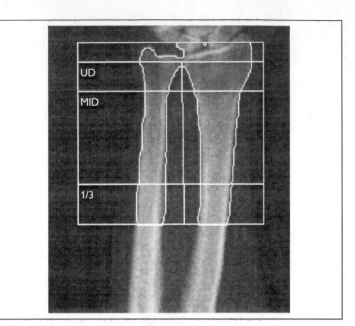

Figure 3.8 Well-Positioned Distal Radius and Ulna.

	BMD (g/cm²)	T-score	Z-score
L₁	1.029	−1.1	−0.4
L₂	1.203	−0.3	0.4
L₃	1.564	2.7	3.4
L₄	1.010	−1.9	−1.2
L₁-L₄	1.113	−0.9	−0.2

	BMD (g/cm²)	T-score	Z-score
L₁	1.028	−1.1	−0.4
L₂	1.210	−0.3	0.4
L₃	1.200	−0.3	0.3
L₄	1.086	−1.3	−0.6
L₁-L₄	1.129	−0.8	−0.1

Figure 3.9 Imaging Studies Interfere with DXA Scans. Imaging Studies at 3 Weeks' Interval. Note Barium in the Colon on the Top Image.

left in a pocket. Similarly, if the patient had a radiological study entailing the intake of radio-opaque material, erroneous results may be obtained (Fig. 3.9). Also, if the patient has taken a calcium tablet before the test is done, the tablet may remain in the vicinity of a vertebra and confound the BMD measurement and T-score calculation.

Pathologies That May Affect the Bone Density

A number of diseases may affect the bone density of individual vertebrae, such as multiple myeloma, Paget's disease of bone, hemangiomas, osteolytic or osteoblastic deposits, previous vertebral fractures, and spine surgery. Vertebral augmentation procedures (e.g., Kyphoplasty, vertebroplasty) result in an increase in BMD.

Vertebral Compression Fractures

When a vertebral fracture occurs, the area of the vertebra is reduced. As there is no change in the amount of mineral in the vertebra, the BMD and T-scores of the affected vertebra are artificially high. The main densitometric features of vertebral compression fractures include (Fig. 3.10):

1. Smaller surface area of the affected vertebra compared with the vertebra immediately above. Typically, the surface area gradually increases from upper to lower lumbar vertebrae.
2. BMD of the affected vertebra is higher than that of the vertebra immediately below it. Normally the BMD gradually increases from upper to lower lumbar vertebrae.
3. A difference in T-scores exceeding 1.0 between the affected vertebra and adjacent vertebrae.

   The diagnosis of vertebral compression fractures can also be established during bone densitometry by the vertebral fracture assessment (VFA), which laterally scans the vertebrae, usually from T4 to the sacrum. The presence of a vertebral compression fracture can be diagnosed by (Fig. 3.11):[3-6]

Noraml lumbar vertebrae			
	Area	BMD	T-score
L1	12.98	1.010	0.8
L2	13.38	1.044	0.1
L3	14.25	1.173	0.8
L4	16.70	1.309	1.8

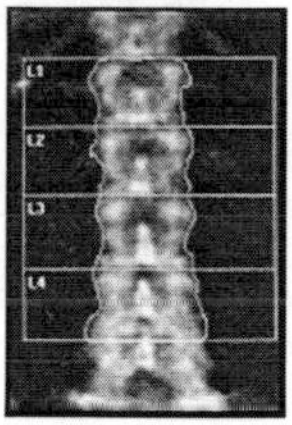

Note:

The gradual increase in area of each vertebra from L1 to L4.

The gradual increase in BMD and BMD from L1 to L4.

The T-score of each vertebra is within 1.0 of the adjacent vertebrae.

Vertebral compression fracture of L2 and L3			
	Area	BMD	T-score
L1	17.20	0.824	−1.7
L2	14.04	1.288	1.8
L3	17.49	1.201	0.9
L4	19.96	1.119	−0.2

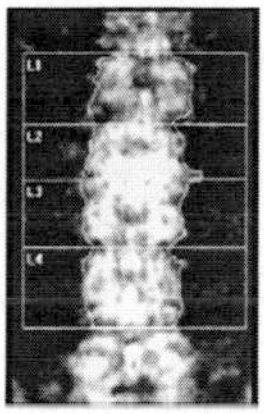

Note:

The heights of L2 and L3 are less than expected.

The BMD of L2 and L3 are higher than L4.

The difference between the T-score of L2 and L3 and adjacent vertebrae is more than 1.0.

Figure 3.10 DXA Findings Suggestive of Vertebral Fractures.

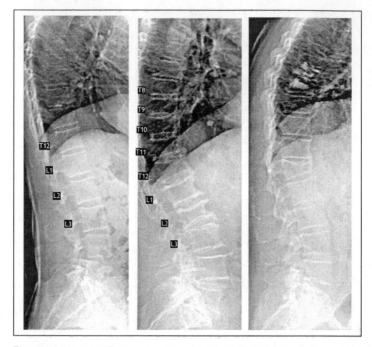

Figure 3.11 Vertebral Fracture Assessment Is Useful to Detect Vertebral Compression Fractures.

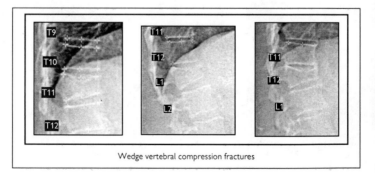

Wedge vertebral compression fractures

Figure 3.12 Different Degrees of Wedge Compression Fractures.

a. Calculating the ratio of the anterior, mid-point, and posterior heights of each vertebra. A vertebral height loss of at least 20%, it is suggestive of a vertebral compression fracture. A software application is available to place markers on the anterior, posterior, and mid-point vertebral heights. The software then calculates the ratio between these heights and those of the adjacent vertebrae to diagnose vertebral compression fractures:

   i. Wedge: if the difference is between the anterior and posterior heights (Fig. 3.12)

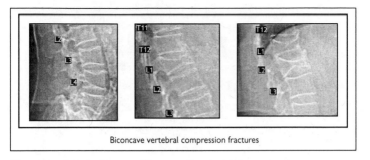

Biconcave vertebral compression fractures

Figure 3.13 Different Degrees of Biconcave Vertebral Compression Fractures.

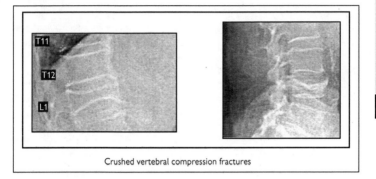

Crushed vertebral compression fractures

Figure 3.14 Crush Vertebrae.

 ii. Biconcave: if the difference is between the mid-point and posterior or anterior height (Fig. 3.13)

 iii. Crush: if the difference is between adjacent vertebral heights (Fig. 3.14)

 b. Visually, by looking at the shape of each vertebra and determining whether it looks "normal" (rectangular in shape) or wedge, biconcave, or crushed.

  The severity is determined according to the ratio of the diameters or visually according to the shape of the vertebrae.

Other Imaging Studies

Plain X-Rays

Experienced radiologists may be able to detect small degrees of bone demineralization on plain x-rays. Untrained eyes, however, can only detect changes of such magnitude of demineralization as to make these observations of little clinical value. Furthermore, changes in exposure, brightness, and contrast may give erroneous impressions about the degree of bone mineralization.

Vertebral compression fractures, however, can be recognized even by relatively inexperienced eyes because the determination of such a fracture is dependent on changes in the shape of the affected vertebra. The same classification system used to diagnose vertebral compression fractures on VFA can be used for the identification of vertebral compression fractures on x-rays.

Quantitative Ultrasound

During quantitative ultrasonography (QUS), a sound wave is generated by a transmitter at one end of the bone studied and the wave is detected by a receiver at the other end of the bone. Two measurements are routinely made: the speed of sound (SOS) and broadband ultrasound attenuation (BUA). The denser the bone, the quicker and less attenuated is the sound wave transmitted. The calcaneus is the bone most studied by QUS.

QUS cannot be used to diagnose osteoporosis using the WHO criteria, cannot be included in the FRAX® algorithm, and is not clinically useful in monitoring the patient's response to therapy.[7]

The portability of QUS devices and their low cost compared with full-body DXA scanners have increased their use. They are often used at health fairs. Population studies have documented a good correlation between calcaneus QUS parameters and fracture risk, including hip fractures.[8,9] QUS devices are sometimes used for epidemiologic studies, but unfortunately their clinical utility is limited.[10] At most, therefore, results of QUS may identify patients at risk of having osteoporosis and fractures.

False-negative results, however, are causes of concern because a patient may have a "normal" calcaneus QUS scan but osteoporosis or osteopenia in the hips or lumbar spine as determined by DXA. Under these circumstances, the patient may receive false reassurance of skeletal health when no such reassurance is warranted. A treatment opportunity will be missed, and the patient subsequently may sustain a fracture that could have been prevented had she been diagnosed and treated for osteoporosis.

Quantitative Computed Tomography

Unlike DXA scanners, which measure the surface area of the bone scanned to calculate its areal BMD (aBMD), quantitative computed tomography (QCT) measures the volume of the bone studied to calculate a volumetric BMD (vBMD). One of the main advantages of QCT is that the measurement can be focused on the body of the vertebra examined and exclude extravertebral calcifications. Consequently, small changes in BMD—such as the ones occurring soon after menopause or when patients are prescribed glucocorticoids—can be readily detected by QCT compared with DXA. Peripheral QCT (pQCT) provides similar information on peripheral bones.

QCT cannot be used to diagnose osteoporosis using the World Health Organization (WHO) criteria and cannot be included in the FRAX® algorithm. Nevertheless, it can be used to estimate fracture risk. Limitations of QCT include the cost of the equipment and expertise needed to operate it and interpret the results. QCT is also much more time consuming than DXA scans, and the patient is exposed to substantial radiation.

Radiogrammetry of the Metacarpal Bones

During radiogrammetry, the bone mass of the middle three metacarpal bones of the nondominant hand is measured by x-ray.[11] The advantages of this method include low cost, low exposure to radiation, and ready availability; it can be performed with conventional radiology or mammography equipment.[12] In localities in which access to DXA is limited, it can be used to identify patients who need a DXA scan.[13]

The International Society for Clinical Densitometry

The ISCD is an international professional society dedicated to ensuring the highest possible standards of bone densitometry and assessment of skeletal health. It educates and certifies clinicians and technologists and accredits DXA facilities. It is a helpful resource for those interested in bone densitometry. A wealth of information is available on its web site: <http://www.iscd.org/>

References

1. Binkley N, Bilezekian JP, Kendler DL, et al. Official Positions of the International Society for Clinical densitometry and Executive Summary of the 2005 Position Development. J Clin Densitom 2006;9:4–14.

2. Federal Guidance Report No 14. Radiation Protection Guidance for Diagnostic and Interventional X-Ray Procedures. 2011. Interagency Working Group on Medical Radiation. US Environmental Protection Agency, Washington, DC 20460.

3. Genant HK, Wu CY, van Kuijk C, et al. Vertebral fracture assessment using a semiquantitative technique. J Bone Miner Res. 1993;8(9):1137–48.

4. Genant HK, Jergas M, Palermo L, et al. Comparison of semiquantitative visual and quantitative morphometric assessment of prevalent and incident vertebral fractures in osteoporosis. J Bone Miner Res. 1996;11(7):984–96.

5. Binkley N, Krueger D, Gangnon R, et al. Lateral vertebral assessment: a valuable technique to detect clinically significant vertebral fractures. Osteoporos Int. 2005;16(12):1513–8.

6. Wu CY, Li J, Jergas M, et al. Comparison of semiquantitative and quantitative techniques for the assessment of prevalent and incident vertebral fractures. Osteoporos Int. 1995;5(5):354–70.

7. Lewiecki EM, Richmond B, Miller PD. Uses and misuses of quantitative ultrasonography in managing osteoporosis. Cleve Clin J Med. 2006;73(8):742–46, 749–52.

8. Siris ES, Miller PD, Barrett-Connor E, et al. Identification and fracture outcomes of undiagnosed low bone mineral density in postmenopausal women: results from the National Osteoporosis Risk Assessment. JAMA. 2001;286(22):2815–22.

9. Moayyeri A, Adams JE, Adler RA, et al. Quantitative ultrasound of the heel and fracture risk assessment: an updated meta-analysis. Osteoporos Int. 2012;23(1):143–53.

10. Pacheco EM, Harrison EJ, Ward KA, et al. Detection of osteoporosis by dual energy X-ray absorptiometry (DXA) of the calcaneus: is the WHO criterion applicable? Calcif Tissue Int. 2002;70(6):475–82.

11. Hyldstrup L, Nielsen SP. Metacarpal index by digital X-ray radiogrammetry: normative reference values and comparison with dual X-ray absorptiometry. J Clin Densitom. 2001;4(4):299–306.

12. Boonen S, Nijs J, Borghs H, et al. Identifying postmenopausal women with osteoporosis by calcaneal ultrasound, metacarpal digital X-ray radiogrammetry and phalangeal radiographic absorptiometry: a comparative study. Osteoporos Int. 2005;16(1):93–100.

13. Dhainaut A, Rohde GE, Syversen U, et al. The ability of hand digital X-ray radiogrammetry to identify middle-aged and elderly women with reduced bone density, as assessed by femoral neck dual-energy X-ray absorptiometry. J Clin Densitom. 2010;13(4):418–25.

Chapter 4

Diagnosis

Goals of the Diagnostic Process

1. Establish the diagnosis and severity.
2. Identify secondary causes (if any) of bone demineralization.
3. Establish a baseline against which the patient's progress can be assessed.

Establishing the Diagnosis of Osteoporosis

Clinical Manifestations

Osteoporosis is clinically silent until the patient sustains a fracture, which is often a catastrophic event that requires immediate medical attention. Vertebral fractures, however, are often silent, and patients may present with loss of height, kyphosis, and gradually worsening back pain. Height loss of more than 2 centimeters over a 3-year period is associated with an increased risk of vertebral fractures (Fig. 4.1).[1]

Fragility fractures, also known as low-trauma, low-energy, or low-impact fractures, are diagnostic of osteoporosis and result from trauma that ordinarily would not be expected to lead to a fracture. A fragility fracture is also defined as a fracture occurring after a fall from a standing position. Fragility fractures can occur spontaneously in the absence of trauma. These atraumatic osteoporotic fractures include previously unsuspected vertebral fractures detected on chest x-rays done for medical conditions unrelated to osteoporosis, or by vertebral imaging techniques such as the vertebral fracture assessment (VFA) performed during dual-energy x-ray absorptiometry (DXA) scans.

Bone Densitometry/Dual-energy X-ray Absorptiometry

Bone densitometry is discussed in Chapter 3. The World Health Organization (WHO) diagnostic criteria are generally accepted worldwide (Fig. 4.2). They are based on the T-score, which is standard deviation difference between the patient's bone mineral density (BMD) compared with that of a young adult

The diagnosis of osteoporosis can be established by:
1. The presence of a fragility fracture,
   OR
2. Bone densitometry: a T-score of -2.5 or lower in the femoral neck, total hip, lumbar vertebrae, or distal one-third radius.

Figure 4.1 The Diagnosis of Osteoporosis.

27

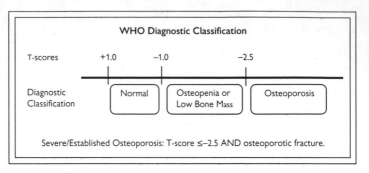

Figure 4.2 World Health Organization Diagnostic Classification for Bone Mass.

sex-matched reference population. The patient has a normal BMD if the T-score is 1.0 or higher, low bone mass (osteopenia) if the T-score is between −1.0 and −2.5, and osteoporosis if the T-score is −2.5 or lower.[2]

The WHO diagnostic guidelines were originally developed based on a postmenopausal white population, but are now used for both genders and other ethnic groups. The cutoff point of −2.5 was selected as it identified the population likely to sustain a fragility fracture. The T-score, as opposed to the Z-score, is used to make the diagnosis of osteoporosis. Although intuitively it may appear more appropriate to compare the patient's BMD to that of an age- and sex-matched population, the patient's BMD should be compared with a reference population in whom the risk of osteoporotic fractures is low so as to identify those more susceptible to fracture.

According to the WHO diagnostic criteria and International Society for Densitometry (ISCD) recommendations, a T-score of −2.5 or lower in any one of the following skeletal sites is consistent with a diagnosis of osteoporosis, provided the quality of the scan is good and there are no artifacts that invalidate the results:[3]

Total Hip/Femoral Neck
Skeletal regions of interest in the hip other than the total hip and femoral neck (e.g., trochanter, Ward's area) should not be used for diagnostic purposes.[4] If both hips are scanned, the lowest value of the two sides should be taken into account, not the mean value.

Lumbar Spine
The L1-L4 T-score should be used, provided there are no artifacts and no evidence of vertebral compression fracture. One or two vertebrae that are invalid for BMD measurement due to a structural abnormality or artifact may be excluded from analysis. A minimum of two lumbar vertebrae should be included in the calculation of the T-score. The ISCD specifically discourages basing the diagnosis on the scan of a single vertebra, known as cherry picking.[4]

When one or more vertebrae are excluded because of vertebral compression fracture, osteophytes, or other artifacts, the ISCD discourages averaging the T-scores of evaluable vertebrae. Most densitometers automatically calculate the T-scores for various combinations of lumbar vertebrae.

> **Only one diagnosis should be made.**
>
> Patients often have densitometric evidence of osteopenia in the femoral neck and osteoporosis in the lumbar vertebrae.
>
> In that instance, the final diagnosis should be "osteoporosis," *not* "osteoporosis of the lumbar vertebrae and osteopenia of the femoral neck."

Figure 4.3 Only One Diagnosis per Patient.

If the BMD and T-score of one vertebra are markedly inconsistent with those of the adjacent vertebrae, causes of localized bone demineralization such as multiple myeloma, hemangiomas, and osteolytic bone deposits or increased calcium deposition such as osteoblastic deposits, Paget's disease of bone, or artifacts should be considered. Vertebral compression fractures may also increase the T-score.

One-Third (1/3) Radius

If neither hip nor lumbar vertebrae scans can be used because the patient's weight exceeds the specifications of the densitometer used—usually about 300 pounds—or because of the presence of artifacts such as bilateral hip replacements, multiple vertebral compression fractures, scoliosis, gross osteophytes, extraosseous calcifications, or postsurgery on the lumbar vertebrae, the ISCD recommends that the forearm be measured. The T-score of the one-third radius, called 1/3 radius on some instruments, may be used for diagnostic classification.[4] Other forearm regions of interest, such as the ultradistal radius, should not be used for diagnosis.

Vertebral Compression Fractures

The presence of a vertebral compression fracture in the absence of significant trauma (fragility fracture) is consistent with a diagnosis of osteoporosis. A vertebral fracture can be identified by imaging such as plain x-rays or VFA, as discussed in Chapter 3.

Other Measurement Technologies

A number of other technologies (e.g., QUS, QCT) are used to measure or estimate BMD. They are briefly discussed in Chapter 3. It is important to recognize that T-scores calculated by non-DXA technologies cannot be used to diagnose osteoporosis using the WHO criteria. The T-score measured by DXA identifies a portion of the population at risk of sustaining a fracture, while the correlation between T-scores measured by other technologies with fracture risk may not be the same, resulting in the over- or under-diagnosis of osteoporosis.

Assessing the Severity of the Condition: Estimating the Fracture Risk

The main purpose of treating osteoporosis is to reduce the fracture risk. Although the WHO diagnostic classification was originally designed to identify patients with osteoporosis but not serve as a treatment guide, it is often used to make therapeutic recommendations. This definition, however, lumps patients who have different fracture risks into the same diagnostic category: patients with T-scores from −1.1 to −2.4 are classified as having osteopenia, and yet the patient with a T-score of −2.4 has a much higher fracture risk than the one with a T-score of −1.1. This classification also does not take into account other factors, apart from BMD, that may affect the fracture risk.

Several tools are available to estimate the fracture risk. The BMD is the single most important factor predicting fractures: the risk of fracture is about doubled for each standard deviation the patient's BMD is below the mean of a young-adult reference population. Several other factors discussed in Chapter 5, however, modulate the risk of fractures and should be taken into consideration when developing a management strategy individualized to the patient's circumstances.

In February 2008, the WHO released the FRAX® tool, a free-of-charge computer-based program to calculate the patient's probability of sustaining a hip or major osteoporotic fracture (i.e., clinical spine, forearm, hip, or shoulder fracture) in the following 10 years. The calculated probability is country-specific, taking into account country-specific fracture data and mortality rates. The input for FRAX® consists of the patient's age, gender, weight, height, and the presence or absence of seven risk factors: a personal history of fractures, a history of hip fracture in one of the biological parents, cigarette smoking, intake of glucocorticoids, rheumatoid arthritis, high alcohol use, secondary osteoporosis, and femoral neck BMD, if available. Fracture probability can be calculated with or without the BMD or T-score of the femoral neck.

Although primarily intended to estimate fracture risk in patients with osteopenia, FRAX® may also be used in patients with osteoporosis to emphasize the increased fracture risk, the seriousness of the disease, and motivate them to comply with therapy.

FRAX® has several benefits compared with the use of relative risk to assess fracture risk; it is individualized to the patient and estimates fracture probability as a percentage. This is readily understood by most patients, who appreciate the severity of their condition and the need to adhere to the prescribed medication. FRAX® has several limitations.[5] First and foremost it does not take into account several risk factors for fractures, especially the patient's propensity to fall[6]—a major contributor to fractures. It also does not take into account several other conditions that increase the risk of falls, including medication such as hypnotics, orthostatic hypotension, or the use of bifocal glasses. All risk factors are addressed in a binary (yes/no) manner,[7–10] FRAX® only takes the BMD of the femoral neck into consideration, not other skeletal sites. It is also not validated for use with patients being treated for osteoporosis, therefore it is usually not advisable for use in monitoring the effects of treatment. Although FRAX® is country-specific, and for the United States is ethnic group–specific (i.e., Caucasian, Black, Hispanic, or Asian), it is not clear how it applies to those who move from one country to another or those of a non-designated or mixed ethnicity.[11] FRAX®, however, is a work in evolution, has undergone several permutations, and the ISCD and International Osteoporosis Foundation have jointly issued official positions providing guidance on the clinical use of FRAX® (Fig. 4.4).[12]

> **How to use the FRAX® program:**
> 1. Open the FRAX® – WHO webpage: <www.shef.ac.uk/FRAX/tool.jsp>
> 2. Click on calculation tab.
> 3. Select continent and country.
> 4. Respond to the various questions.
> 5. Click on "calculate" tab, and the patient's probability of sustaining a hip or major osteoporotic fracture will be displayed.
> 6. Click on the printer icon just above the displayed probability to print the results.

Figure 4.4 Instructions on How to Use FRAX®.

Identifying Secondary Causes of low bone mass

Secondary causes of low bone mass include many disease states and medications (Chapter 5).

Laboratory Work-Up for Osteoporosis

There are no laboratory tests to diagnose osteoporosis or osteopenia. The primary purpose of these tests is to identify secondary causes of low bone mass. Opinions differ on what constitutes the minimum routine laboratory work-up of patients with osteoporosis. The following are generally recommended.

Complete Blood Count

This detects anemia, macrocytosis, and microcytosis, which may suggest nutritional deficiencies, bone marrow infiltration, or other pathologies that may contribute to osteoporosis.

Comprehensive Metabolic Profile

1. Blood urea nitrogen, creatinine, and CO_2 reflect renal function. Impaired renal function may predispose to osteoporosis and osteomalacia and affect the choice of medication. Bisphosphonates should not be administered if the glomerular filtration rate is less than 30 to 35 mL/minute.

2. A moderately elevated alkaline phosphatase in the presence of normal hepatic enzymes may suggest hypovitaminosis D, whereas markedly elevated alkaline phosphatase suggests Paget's disease of the bone or skeletal metastases. A low serum alkaline phosphatase may be seen with malnutrition and hypophosphatasia.

3. An elevated protein level may be caused by multiple myeloma. A decreased protein level may be caused by malnutrition, especially when accompanied by hypoalbuminemia.

4. Serum calcium: as about 50% of the serum calcium is bound to albumin, it is recommended to adjust it for the albumin level before interpreting changes in the serum calcium level. Hypercalcemia suggests primary hyperparathyroidism, underlying neoplastic lesions producing

parathyroid-like hormones, or familial hypocalciuric hypercalcemia (see Chapter 12). Hypocalcemia is suggestive of vitamin D deficiency. In the presence of hypocalcemia, the administration of antiresorptive agents is not recommended because it may acutely worsen the hypocalcemia as a result of the decreased mobilization of calcium from bones to circulation.

Serum 25-hydroxy-vitamin D

To rule out hypovitaminosis D. A low serum vitamin D level impairs the intestinal absorption of vitamin D and may lead to secondary hyperparathyroidism.

Other Tests

1. Serum parathyroid hormone to identify hyperparathyroidism (see Chapter 12).
2. Serum magnesium: a low level interferes with the activity of vitamin D.
3. Serum phosphate: a low serum phosphate level may be caused by a number of conditions, including malnutrition, malabsorption, and excessive phosphate loss, which may be medication induced or secondary to disease states.
4. 24-Hour urinary calcium and sodium excretions: hypercalciuria may induce a negative calcium balance. Causes of hypercalciuria include an excessive sodium intake, hence the need to simultaneously measure the urinary sodium excretion. Loop diuretics increase the renal calcium excretion. Hypercalciuria with no excess sodium excretion tends to occur in families: familial hypercalciuria. A low urinary calcium excretion may be caused by malabsorption.
5. Serum thyroid stimulating hormone (TSH), especially if the patient is on thyroid supplements. A low serum TSH level reflects an excessive, inappropriate dose of thyroid replacement and may lead to bone demineralization. Similarly, patients with hyperthyroidism are more at risk of developing osteoporosis.
6. Antigliadin, anti-endomysial, or tissue transglutaminase antibodies to evaluate for celiac disease if malabsorption is suspected. These patients may have no gastrointestinal symptoms.
7. Serum testosterone in men. The usefulness of this test has been questioned. Although hypogonadism is a recognized cause of low bone mass and osteoporosis in men, there is no compelling reason to assay its serum level unless it is causing symptoms that might require testosterone replacement. Osteoporosis in men is discussed in Chapter 14.

Establishing a Baseline to Monitor the Patient's Progress

DXA Scan

Although a DXA scan is not required to establish the diagnosis of osteoporosis if the patient has sustained a fragility fracture, it is useful to establish a baseline against which the patient's response to treatment can be assessed (see Chapter 9).

Bone Density Imaging Technologies								
	Measure-ment	Dx	Fx Risk Predic-tion	FRAX	Monitor	Cost	Radia-tion	Port-ability
DXA	aBMD	Yes	Yes	Yes	Yes	$$	+	No
pDXA	aBMD	Yes*	Yes	No	No	$	+	Yes
QUS	BUA, SOS	No	Yes	No	No	$	0	Yes
QCT	vBMD	No	Yes	No	Yes	$$$	+++	No
pQCT	vBMD	No	Yes	No	No	$$	++	No

* Only for 33% (1/3) Radius

Figure 4.5 Uses and Limitations of Bone Imaging Studies.

Other Imaging Studies

With the exception of QCT, non-DXA technologies are not clinically useful to monitor changes in BMD (Fig. 4.5).

Laboratory Tests

Markers of bone resorption are useful to determine whether a patient is responding to the prescribed medication (see Chapter 9).

References

1. Siminoski K, Jiang G, Adachi JD, et al. Accuracy of height loss during prospective monitoring for detection of incident vertebral fractures. Osteoporos Int. 2005;16(4):403–10.

2. Kanis JA, Melton LJ 3rd, Christiansen C, et al. The diagnosis of osteoporosis. J Bone Miner Res. 1994;9(8):1137–41.

3. Hans D, Downs RW Jr, Duboeuf F, et al. Skeletal sites for osteoporosis diagnosis: the 2005 ISCD Official Positions. J Clin Densitom. 2006;9(1):15–21.

4. Hamdy RC, Petak SM, Lenchick L, et al. International Society for Clinical densitometry Position Development Panel and Scientific Advisory Committee. Which central DXA skeletal sites and regions of interest should be used to determine the diagnosis of osteoporosis? J Clin Densitom 2002;5(Suppl):S11-S18.

5. Lewiecki EM, Compston JE, Miller PD, et al. Official Positions for FRAX® Bone Mineral Density and FRAX® simplification from Joint Official Positions Development Conference of the International Society for Clinical Densitometry and International Osteoporosis Foundation on FRAX®. J Clin Densitom. 2011;14(3):226–36.

6. Masud T, Binkley N, Boonen S, et al. Official Positions for FRAX® clinical regarding falls and frailty: can falls and frailty be used in FRAX®? From Joint Official Positions Development Conference of the International Society for Clinical Densitometry and International Osteoporosis Foundation on FRAX®. J Clin Densitom. 2011;14(3):194–204.

7. Broy SB, Tanner SB; FRAX(®) Position Development Conference Members. Official Positions for FRAX® clinical regarding rheumatoid arthritis from Joint Official Positions Development Conference of the International Society for Clinical Densitometry and International Osteoporosis Foundation on FRAX®. J Clin Densitom. 2011;14(3):184–9.

8. Blank RD; FRAX(®) Position Development Conference Members. Official Positions for FRAX® clinical regarding prior fractures from Joint Official Positions Development Conference of the International Society for Clinical Densitometry and International Osteoporosis Foundation on FRAX®. J Clin Densitom. 2011;14(3):205–11.

9. Leib ES, Saag KG, Adachi JD, et al. Official Positions for FRAX(®) clinical regarding glucocorticoids: the impact of the use of glucocorticoids on the estimate by FRAX(®) of the 10 year risk of fracture from Joint Official Positions Development Conference of the International Society for Clinical Densitometry and International Osteoporosis Foundation on FRAX(®). J Clin Densitom. 2011;14(3):212–19.

10. Dimai HP, Chandran M; FRAX(®) Position Development Conference Members. Official Positions for FRAX® clinical regarding smoking from Joint Official Positions Development Conference of the International Society for Clinical Densitometry and International Osteoporosis Foundation on FRAX®. J Clin Densitom. 2011;14(3):190–93.

11. Cauley JA, El-Hajj Fuleihan G, Arabi A, et al. Official Positions for FRAX® clinical regarding international differences from Joint Official Positions Development Conference of the International Society for Clinical Densitometry and International Osteoporosis Foundation on FRAX®. J Clin Densitom. 2011;14(3):240–62.

12. Hans DB, Kanis JA, Baim S, et al. Joint Official Positions of the International Society for Clinical Densitometry and International Osteoporosis Foundation on FRAX(®). Executive Summary of the 2010 Position Development Conference on Interpretation and use of FRAX® in clinical practice. J Clin Densitom. 2011;14(3):171–80.

Chapter 5

Identifying Patients at Risk of Fractures

The goal of treating osteoporosis is to prevent fractures. Given the prevalence of osteoporosis, its silent nature until a fracture occurs, the increased risk of re-fracture, and the post-fracture prognosis, patients should ideally be identified and treated before they fracture, and certainly treated after a major low-trauma fracture has occurred. Recommendations and guidelines to screen for osteoporosis[1–6] have been incorporated into the algorithm (Fig. 5.1).[7]

Two separate sets of factors interact to increase fracture risk: bone fragility and propensity to fall. Although some patients fracture spontaneously (atraumatic fractures), in most instances fractures are the result of falls. Awareness of these factors improves the identification of patients at risk of sustaining fractures (Fig. 5.2).

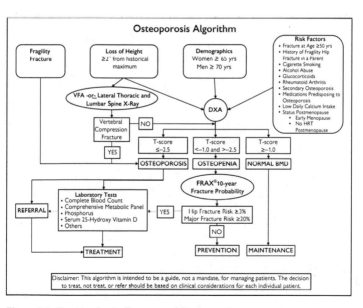

Figure 5.1 Algorithm for the Treatment of Osteoporosis.

Reprinted with permission, Hamdy RC, Baim S, Broy SB, et al. Algorithm for the management of osteoporosis. South Med J. 2010;103(10):1009–15.

(Algorithm for the Management of Osteoporosis. *Southern Medical Journal*, 2010;103(10):1009–17. © 2010 Southern Medical Association. This material is reproduced with the permission of Wolters Kluwer Health.)

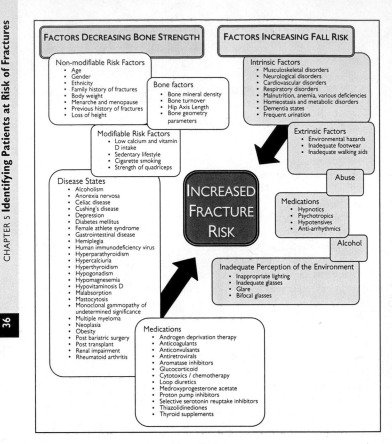

Figure 5.2 Select Factors Affecting Fracture Risk.

Factors Increasing Bone Fragility

Bone Mineral Density

The lower the patient's bone mineral density (BMD), the higher is the fracture risk. There is, however, no threshold; the relationship is exponential.[8] BMD also is not the only factor increasing fracture risk. Many patients with osteoporosis do not sustain fractures and, conversely, many patients with osteopenia, or even normal BMD, sustain fractures.[9] This led to the inclusion of bone quality in the definition of osteoporosis (see Chapter 1).

Bone Turnover

Bone turnover (see Chapter 2) is an independent factor affecting fracture risk.[10,11]

Nonmodifiable Risk Factors

Female Sex

In all ethnic groups women tend to have smaller skeletons than men and are therefore more likely to develop osteoporosis.

Caucasian Ethnicity

White women and men tend to have a smaller skeletal mass than blacks. Ethnic differences in geometry, hip axis length, microarchitecture, and buckling ratio[12,13] may explain ethnic differences in fracture risk (Figs. 5.3 and 5.4).

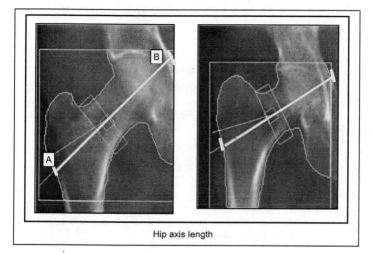

Hip axis length

Figure 5.3 The Hip Axis A Length Affects the Fracture B Risk See text.

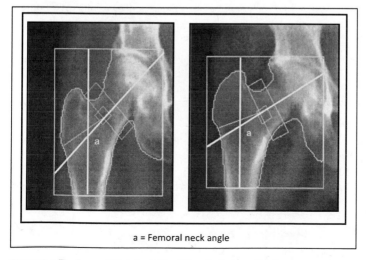

a = Femoral neck angle

Figure 5.4 The Femoral Neck Angle May Affect the Fracture Risk See text.

Hip Axis Length

Hip axis length (HAL), the distance between the inner pelvic brim to the outer edge of the greater trochanter along the femoral neck axis, is a predictor of hip fracture independent of BMD. For each standard deviation increase in HAL, the risk of fracture is almost doubled.[14] Other geometric measurements such as femoral neck-shaft angle and femoral neck width also may affect fracture risk.[15]

Family History of Osteoporosis

A positive family history of osteoporosis—especially fragility hip fracture in one of the biological parents—increases the risk of fractures, particularly hip fractures.[16,17] Several factors predisposing to osteoporosis are not inherited, but are acquired and influenced by the patient's family, such as lifestyle choices.

Aging

Aging is associated with bone loss (see Chapter 2) and is an independent risk factor for fractures.[18] At any given BMD, the fracture risk is higher in older than younger people.[19] Several mechanisms associated with aging lead to a negative calcium balance and predispose to osteoporosis, including reduced physical activity and impaired gastrointestinal absorption of calcium and vitamin D.

Menarche/Menopause

Estrogen exerts a protective effect on the skeleton: It stimulates bone formation and reduces bone resorption. Therefore, a late menarche and early menopause are risk factors for osteoporosis, especially if the menopause is surgical and the patient is not prescribed hormonal replacement therapy. Similarly, patients who have periods of amenorrhea or irregular menstrual cycles are more at risk of low bone mass.

Low Body Weight

A low body weight is an independent predictor of low bone mass and osteoporosis. Women who weigh less than they did when they were 25 years old are more at risk of sustaining fractures.[16,20]

Loss of Height

A historical height loss greater than 1.5 cm is suggestive of vertebral compression fractures.[21] In the absence of significant trauma, these represent fragility fractures, are diagnostic of osteoporosis, and increase the subsequent risk of fractures.

Previous Fragility Fractures

Patients who have sustained fragility fractures are much more at risk of sustaining further fractures.[22]

Modifiable Risk Factors

Whereas genetic factors determine 46% to 62% of BMD, 38% to 54% is determined by lifestyle and environmental factors.[23] Modifiable risk factors leading to low bone mass are discussed in Chapter 6.

Medications Associated with Osteoporosis

A number of medications lead to increased bone fragility and fracture risk (Fig. 5.5).

Medication	Mechanisms/Notes	References
Androgen deprivation therapy	Hypogonadism	24
Anticoagulants	Heparin, not low molecular weight heparin	25
Anticonvulsants	Induction of hepatic enzymes – vitamin D metabolism	26,27
Antiretrovirals	Several mechanisms	28
Aromatase inhibitors	Lowered estrogen levels	29
Cytotoxics/ chemotherapy	Hypogonadism	30
Loop diuretics	Increased renal calcium excretion	31
Medroxyprogesterone acetate	Lowered estrogen levels	32
Proton pump inhibitors	Proton pump inhibitor, not H2 blockers: increased duration-dependent fracture risk	33
Selective serotonin reuptake inhibitors	Negative effect independent of BMD & underlying depression: functional serotonergic pathway in bone cells	34,35
Thiazolidinediones	Dose dependent negative effect on BMD Direct action on bone cell differentiation	36
Thyroid supplements (inappropriate)	Increased bone turnover	37

Figure 5.5 Select Medications Associated with Increased Fracture Risk and/or Decreased BMD/Bone Strength.

Osteoporosis Resulting from Disease States

A number of disease states lead to increased bone fragility and fracture risk (Fig. 5.6).

Factors Increasing the Risk Factors of Falling

Given the precarious equilibrium that allows humans to maintain an upright posture, constantly adjusting to changes in the walking surface and immediate environment, a number of conditions can impair this fragile equilibrium and lead to falls. A discussion of the various causes of falls is beyond the scope of this book. The main purpose of this section is to highlight some causes of falls.

Intrinsic Factors

Musculoskeletal Disorders

The musculoskeletal system provides the framework to maintain an upright posture and locomotion. The instability of the various articulations necessary for proper ambulation is compensated by a well-orchestrated, fine-tuned system of joints, ligaments, muscles, and tendons that allows propulsion while maintaining stability. A fall may result from any disturbance of this fragile equilibrium,

Disease State	Mechanism/Notes	References
Alcoholism	Several mechanisms	38
Anorexia nervosa	Chapter 13	
Celiac disease	Prevalence underestimated because of different degrees	39,40
Cushing's disease	Excess endogenous glucocorticoid production	41
Depression	Possible interference with immune and endocrinal functions	42
Diabetes mellitus	Type 1 and 2, impaired bone quality, increased fracture risk	43,44
	Increased risk of falls: peripheral and autonomic neuropathies, visual impairment, foot problems	
Female athlete syndrome	Chapter 13	
Gastrointestinal diseases	Reduced absorption	45
Hemiplegia	Increased bone demineralization on paralyzed side.	46
	Impaired mobility, increase risk of falls	
Human immunodeficiency virus	Inflammation, infection, hypogonadism, GH deficiency, low body mass index, antiretroviral medications	47
Hyperparathyroidism	Excessive bone resorption; see Chapter 12	48
Hypercalciuria	Negative calcium balance	49,50
Hyperthyroidism	Increased bone turnover rate	51
Hypogonadism	Reduced estrogen levels	52,53
Hypomagnesemia	Often complicates diabetes mellitus and alcoholism	54
Hypovitaminosis D	Decreased intestinal calcium absorption, negative calcium balance, hyperparathyroidism	Chapters 2 & 6
Malabsorption	Negative calcium balance, nutritional deficiencies	55
Mastocytosis	Excessive products of mast cells degranulation promote osteoclast differentiation. Increased bone resorption	56
Monoclonal gammopathy of undetermined significance	Activation of osteoclasts	57
Multiple myeloma	Activation of osteoclasts, hypercalcemia, glucocorticoid administration, chemotherapy	58
Neoplasia	Parathyroid-like hormone, loss of appetite, chemotherapy, radiation therapy	59
Obesity	Increased adiposity associated with hypovitaminosis D and secondary hyperparathyroidism	60,61

Figure 5.6 Select Disease States Associated with Increased Bone Fragility and/or Decreased BMD/Bone Strength, Alphabetically Arranged.

Disease State	Mechanism/Notes	References
Post bariatric surgery	Weight loss, malabsorption	62,63
Post-transplant	Underlying condition, glucocorticoid and immunosuppressants	64
Renal impairment	Impaired activation of vitamin D, acidosis.	65
Rheumatoid arthritis	Pro-inflammatory cytokine milieu increases bone resorption	66,67
	Medications used	
	Reduced physical capabilities, increased fall risk	

Figure 5.6 (Continued)

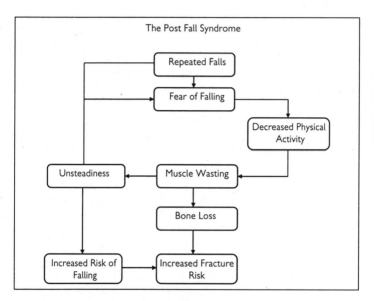

Figure 5.7 The Vicious Cycle of Falls and Fractures.

including degenerative and inflammatory arthropathies, fractures, ligamentous damage, myopathies, and sarcopenia.

Some patients who fall are so afraid of sustaining more falls that they restrict their physical activities and spend most of the time sedentary: the post-fall syndrome. This triggers a vicious circle: Less physical activity leads to gradual muscle wasting, which in turn leads to bone demineralization and increased fragility of the skeleton. Reduced physical activity also leads to unsteadiness and increases the risk of falls, further increasing the risk of fractures (Fig. 5.7).

Neurologic Disorders

The nervous system integrates various stimuli received from receptors, and by contracting and relaxing various muscle groups maintains an upright stable posture, allows safe ambulation, and prevents falls. Any interference with the proper functioning of the central or peripheral nervous system may predispose to falls, including peripheral neuropathies, spinal cord injuries, cerebrovascular accidents/strokes, epilepsy, Parkinson's disease, and other diseases associated with involuntary movements, space-occupying lesions, and hydrocephalus.

Cardiovascular Disorders

The cardiovascular system maintains an adequate blood supply to the brain, which has no reserve capacity and therefore is dependent on blood circulation to meet its needs. Unsteadiness and falls may result from interference with cerebral/cerebellar blood flow, such as postural/orthostatic hypotension, arrhythmias, sensitive carotid sinus, vertebrobasilar insufficiency, transient ischemic attacks, and low fixed cardiac output.

Frequent Urination

Frequent urination and erectile dysfunction are associated with an increased fracture risk.[68]

Respiratory Disorders

Although respiratory causes are rarely direct causes of falls, dyspnea and coughing may induce falls by taxing the precarious equilibrium maintaining balance and an upright posture.

Malnutrition, Anemia, and Various Deficiencies

An adequate nutritional state is necessary to optimize the body's physical functioning. Nutritional deficiencies may cause myopathies and muscle wasting.

Homeostasis and Metabolic Disorders

Diabetes mellitus is often complicated by peripheral and autonomic neuropathies, which predispose to falls. Type 1 and type 2 diabetes mellitus are both risk factors for fracture. Hepatic or renal impairment, although not directly contributing to falls, may increase the individual's propensity to fall.

Dementing illnesses

Patients with dementia are at risk of falling because they may not be aware of the hazards associated with some of their activities and because of their easy distractibility. Patients with Lewy body dementia and Parkinson's disease dementia also have tremors and neurologic deficits that may increase the risk of falls.

Medications

Any medication interfering with equilibrium, cognition, and level of consciousness may disrupt the physical equilibrium and blunt postural reflexes, increasing the risk of falls. This is particularly of concern in older people, as the metabolic degradation of most medications is slower than in younger people, resulting in a longer half-life that may lead to drug accumulation. Alcohol potentiates the effect of many psychotropic agents and increases the risk of falls.

Extrinsic and Environmental Factors

Environmental Hazards

Inadequate lighting, glare, small loose rugs, trailing wires, unfamiliar surroundings, and low-lying obstacles may increase the likelihood of tripping and falling.

Inadequate Footwear and Walking Aids

Inappropriate footwear may reduce stability and predispose to falls. Similarly, too short or too high canes or walking aids may interfere with the person's equilibrium and lead to falls. Canes or other walking aids should not be used without consulting a professional health care provider experienced in that area.

Abuse

In the absence of hard data it is difficult to ascertain how many falls can be attributed to physical abuse, which can be by omission or commission.

Impaired Perception of the Environment

If the patient is not able to accurately perceive her environment, she may not be able to avoid hazards in her way, and may trip and fall. Cataracts, glaucoma, macular degeneration, and inadequate glasses may increase the risk of falls. Bifocal eyeglasses are particularly hazardous, because the lower lens, which is meant for near vision, is used to perceive the area immediately surrounding the feet, which therefore can appear distorted, thus increasing the risk of falls. This is especially the case while negotiating stairs (Fig. 5.8).

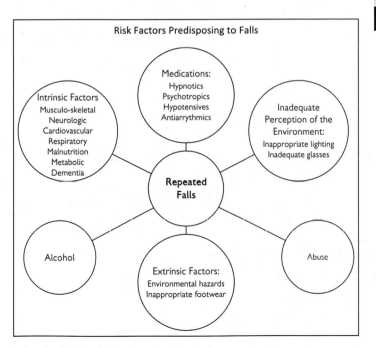

Figure 5.8 Select Risk Factors Predisposing to Falls.

Management of Fractures

Unfortunately, the availability of medications to significantly reduce the risk of further fractures and the progress and innovations in orthopedic surgery witnessed over the past few years have not been matched by an overall improvement in treatment to reduce the risk of future fractures. Many patients who sustain osteoporotic fractures are still neither diagnosed nor treated for osteoporosis. This is regrettable, because the patient is more likely to adhere to a medication regimen if it is started as part of the fracture management program rather than weeks or months later. The availability of parenterally administered medications diminishes compliance issues and the risedronate extended-release formulation simplifies the routine of taking oral bisphosphonates.

The American Orthopedic Association launched the "Own the Bone Program" specifically to this effect, and many institutions have their own algorithms and comprehensive fracture management programs to address this issue, but there is still much to be done to ensure that patients who have sustained osteoporotic fractures and therefore are at risk of further fractures are treated for osteoporosis. The means to reduce fractures are available and effective; unfortunately, they are not used to their fullest extent.

References

1. U.S. Preventive Services Task Force. Screening for Osteoporosis: U.S. Preventive Services Task Force Recommendation Statement. Ann Intern Med 2011;154:356–64.

2. Lim LS, Hoeksema LJ, Sherin K, et al. Screening for osteoporosis in the adult U.S. population: ACPM position statement on preventive practice. Am J Prev Med. 2009;36(4):366–75.

3. Compston J, Cooper A, Cooper C, et al. Guidelines for the diagnosis and management of osteoporosis in postmenopausal women and men from the age of 50 years in the UK. Maturitas. 2009;62(2):105–08.

4. Qaseem A, Snow V, Shekelle P, et al. Screening for osteoporosis in men: a clinical practice guideline from the American College of Physicians. Ann Intern Med. 2008;148(9):680–84.

5. Watts NB, Lewiecki EM, Miller PD, et al. National Osteoporosis Foundation 2008 Clinician's Guide to Prevention and Treatment of Osteoporosis and the World Health Organization Fracture Risk Assessment Tool (FRAX): what they mean to the bone densitometrist and bone technologist. J Clin Densitom. 2008;11(4):473–77.

6. Papaioannou A, Morin S, Cheung AM, et al. 2010 clinical practice guidelines for the diagnosis and management of osteoporosis in Canada: summary. CMAJ. 2010;182(17):1864–73.

7. Hamdy RC, Baim S, Broy SB, et al. Algorithm for the management of osteoporosis. South Med J. 2010;103(10):1009–15.

8. Marshall D, Johnell O, Wedel H. Meta-analysis of how well measures of bone mineral density predict occurrence of osteoporotic fractures. BMJ. 1996;312(7041):1254–59.

9. Siris ES, Chen YT, Abbott TA, et al. Bone mineral density thresholds for pharmacological intervention to prevent fractures. Arch Intern Med. 2004;164(10):1108–12.

10. Unnanuntana A, Gladnick BP, Donnelly E, et al. The assessment of fracture risk. J Bone Joint Surg Am. 2010;92(3):743–53.

11. Chapurlat RD, Garnero P, Bréart G, et al. Serum type I collagen breakdown product (serum CTX) predicts hip fracture risk in elderly women: the EPIDOS study. Bone. 2000;27(2):283–86.

12. Cummings SR, Cauley JA, Palermo L, et al. Racial differences in hip axis lengths might explain racial differences in rates of hip fracture. Study of Osteoporotic Fractures Research Group. Osteoporos Int. 1994;4(4):226–29.

13. Kim KM, Brown JK, Kim KJ, et al. Differences in femoral neck geometry associated with age and ethnicity. Osteoporos Int. 2011;22(7):2165–74.

14. Faulkner KG, Cummings SR, Black D, et al. Simple measurement of femoral geometry predicts hip fracture: the study of osteoporotic fractures. J Bone Miner Res. 1993;8(10):1211–17.

15. Bonnick SL. Bone densitometry in clinical practice: application and interpretation. 2nd ed. Totowa, NJ: Humana Press; 2004.

16. Cummings SR, Nevitt MC, Browner WS, et al. Risk factors for hip fracture in white women. Study of Osteoporotic Fractures Research Group. N Engl J Med. 1995;332(12):767–73.

17. Kanis JA, Borgstrom F, De Laet C, et al. Assessment of fracture risk. Osteoporos Int. 2005;16(6):581–89.

18. Siris ES, Brenneman SK, Barrett-Connor E, et al. The effect of age and bone mineral density on the absolute, excess, and relative risk of fracture in postmenopausal women aged 50–99: results from the National Osteoporosis Risk Assessment (NORA). Osteoporos Int. 2006;17(4):565–74.

19. Hui SL, Slemenda CW, Johnston CC Jr. Age and bone mass as predictors of fracture in a prospective study. J Clin Invest. 1988;81(6):1804–09.

20. Chapurlat RD, Bauer DC, Nevitt M, et al. Incidence and risk factors for a second hip fracture in elderly women. The Study of Osteoporotic Fractures. Osteoporos Int. 2003;14(2):130–36.

21. Bennani L, Allali F, Rostom S, et al. Relationship between historical height loss and vertebral fractures in postmenopausal women. Clin Rheumatol. 2009;28(11):1283–89.

22. Kanis JA, Johnell O, De Laet C, et al. A meta-analysis of previous fracture and subsequent fracture risk. Bone. 2004;35(2):375–82.

23. Body JJ, Bergmann P, Boonen S, et al. Non-pharmacological management of osteoporosis: a consensus of the Belgian Bone Club. Osteoporos Int. 2011;22(11):2769–88.

24. Smith MR, Lee WC, Brandman J, et al. Gonadotropin-releasing hormone agonists and fracture risk: a claims-based cohort study of men with nonmetastatic prostate cancer. J Clin Oncol. 2005;23(31):7897–903.

25. Carlin AJ, Farquharson RG, Quenby SM, et al. Prospective observational study of bone mineral density during pregnancy: low molecular weight heparin versus control. Hum Reprod. 2004;19(5):1211–14.

26. Ensrud KE, Walczak TS, Blackwell TL, et al. Antiepileptic drug use and rates of hip bone loss in older men: a prospective study. Neurology. 2008;71(10):723–30.

27. Pack AM, Morrell MJ, Randall A, et al. Bone health in young women with epilepsy after one year of antiepileptic drug monotherapy. Neurology. 2008;70(18):1586–93.

28. Brown TT, Qaqish RB. Antiretroviral therapy and the prevalence of osteopenia and osteoporosis: a meta-analytic review. AIDS. 2006;20(17):2165–74.

29. Coleman RE, Banks LM, Girgis SI, et al. Skeletal effects of exemestane on bone-mineral density, bone biomarkers, and fracture incidence in postmenopausal women with early breast cancer participating in the Intergroup Exemestane Study (IES): a randomised controlled study. Lancet Oncol. 2007;8(2):119–27.

30. Molina JR, Barton DL, Loprinzi CL. Chemotherapy-induced ovarian failure: manifestations and management. Drug Saf. 2005;28(5):401–16.

31. Lim LS, Fink HA, Kuskowski MA, et al. Loop diuretic use and increased rates of hip bone loss in older men: the Osteoporotic Fractures in Men Study. Arch Intern Med. 2008;168(7):735–40.

32. Guilbert ER, Brown JP, Kaunitz AM, et al. The use of depot-medroxyprogesterone acetate in contraception and its potential impact on skeletal health. Contraception. 2009;79(3):167–77.

33. Roux C, Briot K, Gossec L, et al. Increase in vertebral fracture risk in postmenopausal women using omeprazole. Calcif Tissue Int. 2009;84(1):13–19.

34. Wu Q, Bencaz AF, Hentz JG, et al. Selective serotonin reuptake inhibitor treatment and risk of fractures: a meta-analysis of cohort and case-control studies. Osteoporos Int. 2012;23(1):365–75.

35. Pitts CJ, Kearns AE. Update on medications with adverse skeletal effects. Mayo Clin Proc. 2011;86(4):338–43.

36. Meier C, Kraenzlin ME, Bodmer M, et al. Use of thiazolidinediones and fracture risk. Arch Intern Med. 2008;168(8):820–25.

37. Stein E, Shane E. Secondary osteoporosis. Endocrinol Metab Clin North Am. 2003;32(1):115–34, vii.

38. Maurel DB, Boisseau N, Benhamou CL, et al. Alcohol and bone: review of dose effects and mechanisms. Osteoporos Int. 2012;23(1):1–16.

39. Stenson WF, Newberry R, Lorenz R, et al. Increased prevalence of celiac disease and need for routine screening among patients with osteoporosis. Arch Intern Med. 2005;165(4):393–99.

40. Bianchi ML, Bardella MT. Bone in celiac disease. Osteoporos Int. 2008;19(12):1705–16.

41. Hadjidakis D, Tsagarakis S, Roboti C, et al. Does subclinical hypercortisolism adversely affect the bone mineral density of patients with adrenal incidentalomas? Clin Endocrinol (Oxf). 2003;58(1):72–77.

42. Cizza G. Major depressive disorder is a risk factor for low bone mass, central obesity, and other medical conditions. Dialogues Clin Neurosci. 2011;13(1):73–87.

43. Räkel A, Sheehy O, Rahme E, et al. Osteoporosis among patients with type 1 and type 2 diabetes. Diabetes Metab. 2008;34(3):193–205.

44. Hofbauer LC, Brueck CC, Singh SK, et al. Osteoporosis in patients with diabetes mellitus. J Bone Miner Res. 2007;22(9):1317–28.

45. Bernstein CN, Leslie WD, Leboff MS. AGA technical review on osteoporosis in gastrointestinal diseases. Gastroenterology. 2003;124(3):795–841.

46. Hamdy RC, Moore SW, Cancellaro VA, et al. Long-term effects of strokes on bone mass. Am J Phys Med Rehabil. 1995;74(5):351–56.

47. Triant VA, Brown TT, Lee H, et al. Fracture prevalence among human immunodeficiency virus (HIV)-infected versus non-HIV-infected patients in a large U.S. healthcare system. J Clin Endocrinol Metab. 2008;93(9):3499–504.

48. Bilezikian JP, Khan AA, Potts JT Jr; Third International Workshop on the Management of Asymptomatic Primary Hyperthyroidism. Guidelines for the management of asymptomatic primary hyperparathyroidism: summary

statement from the third international workshop. J Clin Endocrinol Metab. 2009;94(2):335–39.

49. Sakhaee K, Maalouf NM, Kumar R, et al. Nephrolithiasis-associated bone disease: pathogenesis and treatment options. Kidney Int. 2011;79(4):393–403.

50. Garc'a-Nieto V, Navarro JF, Monge M, et al. Bone mineral density in girls and their mothers with idiopathic hypercalciuria. Nephron Clin Pract. 2003;94(4):c89–93.

51. Bassett JH, O'Shea PJ, Srlskantharajah S, et al. Thyroid hormone excess rather than thyrotropin deficiency induces osteoporosis in hyperthyroidism. Mol Endocrinol. 2007;21(5):1095–107.

52. Ebeling PR. Clinical practice. Osteoporosis in men. N Engl J Med. 2008;358(14):1474–82.

53. Khosla S, Amin S, Orwoll E. Osteoporosis in men. Endocr Rev. 2008;29(4):441–64.

54. Fatemi S, Ryzen E, Flores J, et al. Effect of experimental human magnesium depletion on parathyroid hormone secretion and 1,25-dihydroxyvitamin D metabolism. J Clin Endocrinol Metab. 1991;73(5):1067–72.

55. Harpavat M, Keljo DJ, Regueiro MD. Metabolic bone disease in inflammatory bowel disease. J Clin Gastroenterol. 2004;38(3):218–24.

56. Chiappetta N, Gruber B. The role of mast cells in osteoporosis. Semin Arthritis Rheum. 2006;36(1):32–36.

57. Abrahamsen B, Andersen I, Christensen SS, et al. Utility of testing for monoclonal bands in serum of patients with suspected osteoporosis: retrospective, cross sectional study. BMJ. 2005;330(7495):818.

58. Melton LJ 3rd, Kyle RA, Achenbach SJ, et al. Fracture risk with multiple myeloma: a population-based study. J Bone Miner Res. 2005;20(3):487–93.

59. Barton BE. Interleukin-6 and new strategies for the treatment of cancer, hyperproliferative diseases and paraneoplastic syndromes. Expert Opin Ther Targets. 2005;9(4):737–52.

60. Compston JE, Watts NB, Chapurlat R, et al. Obesity is not protective against fracture in postmenopausal women: GLOW. Am J Med. 2011;124(11):1043–50.

61. Premaor MO, Pilbrow L, Tonkin C, et al. Obesity and fractures in postmenopausal women. J Bone Miner Res. 2010;25(2):292–97.

62. Fleischer J, Stein EM, Bessler M, et al. The decline in hip bone density after gastric bypass surgery is associated with extent of weight loss. J Clin Endocrinol Metab. 2008;93(10):3735–40.

63. Wang A, Powell A. The effects of obesity surgery on bone metabolism: what orthopedic surgeons need to know. Am J Orthop (Belle Mead NJ). 2009;38(2):77–79.

64. Ebeling PR. Approach to the patient with transplantation-related bone loss. J Clin Endocrinol Metab. 2009;94(5):1483–90.

65. Jamal SA, Swan VJ, Brown JP, et al. Kidney function and rate of bone loss at the hip and spine: the Canadian Multicentre Osteoporosis Study. Am J Kidney Dis. 2010;55(2):291–99.

66. Ghazi M, Kolta S, Briot K, et al. Prevalence of vertebral fractures in patients with rheumatoid arthritis: revisiting the role of glucocorticoids. Osteoporos Int. 2012;23(2):581–87.

67. Hofbauer LC, Hamann C, Ebeling PR. Approach to the patient with secondary osteoporosis. Eur J Endocrinol. 2010;162(6):1009–20.

68. Frost M, Abrahamsen B, Masud T, et al. Risk factors for fracture in elderly men: a population-based prospective study. Osteoporos Int. 2012;23(2):521–31.

Chapter 6

Nonpharmacologic Management of Osteopenia and Osteoporosis

A number of nonpharmacologic strategies improve skeletal health and enhance the effect of prescribed medications for low bone mass. On their own, these strategies are not sufficient to treat osteoporosis, but in conjunction with anti-resorptives or osteoanabolics, can improve clinical outcomes.

Nutrition

Adequate Daily Calcium and Vitamin D Intake

An adequate daily calcium and vitamin D intake is a sine qua non for bone health and optimal response to the prescribed medication.[1] The Institute of Medicine (IOM) recommendations issued in November 2010 are shown in the accompanying table (Fig. 6.1). These recommendations challenge the concept that "more is better" and instead promote the concept that too much may be harmful. Adverse outcomes of excess calcium and vitamin D intake include hypercalcemia, hypercalciuria, vascular and soft tissue calcification,

Age group (years)	Calcium		Vitamin D	
	RDA+ mg/day	ULI++ mg/day	RDA IU/day	ULI IU/day
1–3	700	2,500	600	2,500
4–8	1,000	2,500	600	3,000
9–18	1,300	3,000	600	4,000
19–30	1,000	2,500	600	4,000
19–50	1,000	2,500	600	4,000
51–70 males	1,000	2,000	600	4,000
51–70 females	1,200	2,000	600	4,000
>70 years	1,200	2,000	800	4,000

+ Recommended Dietary Allowance

++ Upper Level Intake

Figure 6.1 Institute of Medicine Guidelines, November 2010.

Adapted from Institute of Medicine (US) Committee to Review Dietary Reference Intakes for Vitamin D and Calcium; Ross AC, Taylor CL, Yaktine AL, et al. Dietary Reference Intakes for Calcium and Vitamin D. Washington (DC): National Academies Press (US); 2011.

nephrolithiasis, constipation, and interactions with iron and zinc.[2] The IOM also considers a serum 25-hydroxy-vitamin D level of 20 ng/mL (50 nmol/L) as sufficient.[3] Some clinicians, scientists, and societies disagree with this report. The National Osteoporosis Foundation recommends that adults under the age of 50 years have a total daily intake of 1,000 mg of calcium and 400 to 800 international units (IU) of vitamin D. For those aged 50 years and older, the recommended daily intake is 1,200 mg of calcium and 800 to 1,000 IU vitamin D.[4]

Patients with hyperlipidemia or coronary artery disease are often reluctant to consume dairy products because of concerns about raising their serum lipid levels. Nonfat or low-fat dairy products, however, contain an equal, or slightly higher, amount of calcium compared with full-fat products. Similarly, patients with renal calculi often refrain from consuming calcium-containing food. Optimizing daily dietary calcium intake may actually reduce the risk of renal calculi. Red meat (high sulfur-containing amino acids), salt, and caffeine on the other hand increase the urinary calcium excretion. The intake of calcium supplements may increase the risk of renal calculi. Vitamin D and calcium metabolism are discussed in Chapters 2 and 4.

A Well-Balanced, Adequate Diet

A well-balanced diet is important for optimum bone health.[5] Undernutrition, malnutrition, and traditional diets may have negative impacts on skeletal mass.[6] A low protein intake is associated with an increased risk of hip fractures.[7] Vegetarians are not, however, at an increased risk of sustaining fractures.[8] Dairy products rich in calcium, proteins, phosphorus, and potassium are ideal for maintaining calcium homeostasis and bone health.

Avoid Excessive Salt Intake

Excessive salt intake increases renal calcium excretion and may induce a negative calcium balance and bone demineralization.[8] Excessive sodium intake can be through the voluntary addition of salt to food, the use of large amounts of salt while cooking, or the use of preserved and fast food.

Avoid Excessive Caffeine Intake

Excessive caffeine intake increases renal calcium excretion and may lead to a negative calcium balance. The daily consumption of more than 2.5 cups of coffee or 5 cups of tea over a 2-year period was associated with an increased risk of hip fracture in the Framingham Study.[9]

Avoid Excessive Carbonated Soda Beverages

Some carbonated soda beverages may have a negative impact on bone mass:[10] Sodium and caffeine increase renal calcium excretion, whereas phosphoric acid binds to calcium in the gastrointestinal track and reduces its absorption. Perhaps the main concern with high intake of these beverages is the displacement of beneficial liquids, such as milk.

Lifestyle Changes

Avoid or Discontinue Cigarette Smoking

Cigarette smoking increases the risk of osteoporosis and fractures.[11] The effect of cigarette smoking on bone mass during the growth period cannot be reversed once peak bone mass is reached. Notwithstanding, discontinuing cigarette smoking reduces the rate of bone demineralization in all age groups.

Avoid or Discontinue Alcohol Abuse

Whereas low to moderate alcohol consumption (i.e., one drink a day for women and two drinks a day for men) may be beneficial to bone tissue, consumption of four or more drinks a day for men and two or more for women is deleterious to the skeleton and increases the risk of fractures.[6] Alcohol has direct effects on osteoclasts, osteoblasts, and osteocytes, interferes with mechanisms controlling the activity of these cells, and exerts indirect effects through calorie intake, nutritional deficiencies, homeostatic changes, and changes in body composition.[12] The risk of falls is also increased in alcohol abusers.

Physical Exercise

Physical exercise affects bone health by increasing bone mass and reducing the risk of falls, thereby potentially reducing the risk of fractures. Unfortunately, most studies on the effect of physical exercise do not have fractures as an endpoint.[8] Lack of physical exercise and sedentary lifestyles are associated with a smaller bone mass and therefore increased susceptibility to osteoporosis. Conversely, physical exercise is associated with increased muscle and bone mass.[13–15] Several studies documented the positive effects of walking, aerobics, Tai Chi, and resistance exercises on bone mass and density in various age groups and the positive effects of physical exercise on balance, gait, muscle strength, walking speed, and physical performance in older subjects.[8,16,17]

For those interested and able to exercise, general recommendations include exercising for 15 to 60 minutes two to three times a week doing a combination of aerobic exercises and resistance exercises at 70% to 80% of maximum strength.[8] The usual precautions should be observed while prescribing exercises to older patients who have not exercised regularly. Start at a low level, gradually increase duration and intensity of exercise, reduce pace or stop if feeling dizzy, breathless, unsteady, in pain, or experiencing palpitations. Ensure adequate warm-up and cool-down periods. Supervision during the first sessions may be recommended for those leading sedentary lifestyles. An experienced physical therapist or trainer may help develop an individualized exercise program tailored to specific needs of patients with osteoporosis.

Fall Prevention

The prevalence of falls increases with age. About one-third of community-dwelling people over the age of 65 years sustain at least one fall a year, and 5% to 10% of falls result in fractures.[18] The morbidity associated with falls is significant. The adequate management of falls in older people requires the collaboration of a dedicated team to evaluate the patient's medical condition, psychosocial background and medications to develop a management strategy geared to the patient's individual circumstances. Common causes of falls are discussed in Chapter 5.

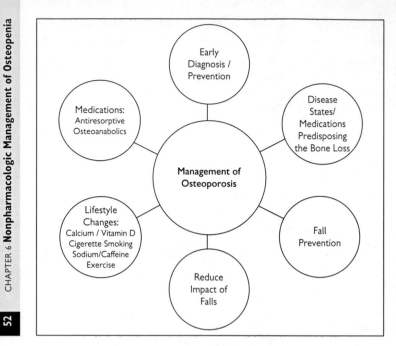

Figure 6.2 The Multiple Facets of Managing Osteoporosis.

Reducing the Impact of Falls: Hip Protectors

If falls cannot be prevented, their consequences may be reduced by providing padding to dissipate the trauma, divert it from bone to adjacent soft tissues, and reduce the risk of fracture. Several hip protectors are commercially available. Studies assessing the efficacy of hip protectors yielded mixed results.[8] Compliance is a major problem: Many patients are reluctant or forget to wear them. Hip protectors are only effective if worn by the patient (Fig. 6.2).

References

1. Body JJ, Bergmann P, Boonen S, et al. Evidence-based guidelines for the pharmacological treatment of postmenopausal osteoporosis: a consensus document by the Belgian Bone Club. Osteoporos Int. 2010;21(10):1657–80.

2. Body JJ, Bergmann P, Boonen S, et al. Extraskeletal benefits and risks of calcium, vitamin D and anti-osteoporosis medications. Osteoporos Int. 2012;23 Suppl 1:S1–23.

3. Institute of Medicine (US) Committee to Review Dietary Reference Intakes for Vitamin D and Calcium; Ross AC, Taylor CL, Yaktine AL, et al. Dietary Reference Intakes for Calcium and Vitamin D. Washington (DC): National Academies Press (US); 2011.

4. National Osteoporosis Foundation. Calcium: What You Should Know. Available at: http://www.nof.org/aboutosteoporosis/prevention/calcium. Accessibility verified March 27, 2012.

5. Rivlin RS. Keeping the young-elderly healthy: is it too late to improve our health through nutrition? Am J Clin Nutr. 2007;86(5):1572S-6S.

6. Fairweather-Tait SJ, Skinner J, Guile GR, et al. Diet and bone mineral density study in postmenopausal women from the TwinsUK registry shows a negative association with a traditional English dietary pattern and a positive association with wine. Am J Clin Nutr. 2011;94(5):1371–75.

7. Munger RG, Cerhan JR, Chiu BC. Prospective study of dietary protein intake and risk of hip fracture in postmenopausal women. Am J Clin Nutr. 1999;69(1):147–52.

8. Body JJ, Bergmann P, Boonen S, et al. Non-pharmacological management of osteoporosis: a consensus of the Belgian Bone Club. Osteoporos Int. 2011;22(11):2769–88.

9. Kiel DP, Felson DT, Hannan MT, et al. Caffeine and the risk of hip fracture: the Framingham Study. Am J Epidemiol. 1990;132(4):675–84.

10. Tucker KL, Morita K, Qiao N, et al. Colas, but not other carbonated beverages, are associated with low bone mineral density in older women: The Framingham Osteoporosis Study. Am J Clin Nutr. 2006;84(4):936–42.

11. Yan C, Avadhani NG, Iqbal J. The effects of smoke carcinogens on bone. Curr Osteoporos Rep. 2011;9(4):202–09.

12. Maurel DB, Boisseau N, Benhamou CL, et al. Alcohol and bone: review of dose effects and mechanisms. Osteoporos Int. 2012;23(1):1–16.

13. Nikander R, Sievänen H, Heinonen A, et al. Targeted exercise against osteoporosis: A systematic review and meta-analysis for optimising bone strength throughout life. BMC Med. 2010;8:47–63.

14. Howe TE, Shea B, Dawson LJ, et al. Exercise for preventing and treating osteoporosis in postmenopausal women. Cochrane Database Syst Rev. 2011 Jul 6;(7):CD000333.

15. Langsetmo L, Hitchcock CL, Kingwell EJ, et al. Physical activity, body mass index and bone mineral density-associations in a prospective population-based cohort of women and men: the Canadian Multicentre Osteoporosis Study (CaMos). Bone. 2012;50(1):401–08.

16. Wayne PM, Kiel DP, Krebs DE, et al. The effects of Tai Chi on bone mineral density in postmenopausal women: a systematic review. Arch Phys Med Rehabil. 2007;88(5):673–80.

17. de Kam D, Smulders E, Weerdesteyn V, et al. Exercise interventions to reduce fall-related fractures and their risk factors in individuals with low bone density: a systematic review of randomized controlled trials. Osteoporos Int. 2009;20(12):2111–25.

18. Masud T, Morris RO. Epidemiology of falls. Age Ageing. 2001;30 Suppl 4:3–7.

Chapter 7

Pharmacologic Management of Osteoporosis, Part 1

The goal of treating osteoporosis is to reduce fracture risk. The final decision as to whom, when, and how to treat is made by the treating clinician in conjunction with the patient, taking into consideration bone mineral density (BMD), risk factors predisposing to fractures and falls, as well as the patient's overall condition. This decision cannot and should not be based solely on the results of a test or score, but is modulated by the clinician's personal experience and the individual circumstances of the patient (Fig. 7.1).

In the United States, the National Osteoporosis Foundation (NOF) guidelines recommend treating patients who have osteoporosis as determined by bone densitometry or the presence of fragility fractures. The guidelines also recommend treating patients who have osteopenia if their probability of sustaining a fracture in the next 10 years as determined by the World Health Organization FRAX® (Fracture Risk Assessment) tool is or exceeds 3% or 20% for hip or major osteoporotic fractures (i.e., clinical spine, forearm, hip or shoulder fracture), respectively.

For patients who have osteopenia and whose FRAX® scores do not reach the threshold recommended by the NOF to initiate treatment, the main goal is to prevent, as opposed to treat, osteoporosis. Although many medications used for the treatment of osteoporosis are the same as those used for prevention, the dosage is sometimes different.

The decision to treat or not to treat should be based on the patient's overall condition and circumstances, and not only on FRAX® or T-scores.

Three different scenarios are presented. All are 66-year-old Caucasian women with a T-score of −1.8 and FRAX® scores of 2.1% and 17% for the probabilities of sustaining hip and major osteoporotic fractures, respectively.

Mrs. LB is on no medication, leads a physically active lifestyle, and exercises regularly. She has not had any fall. The goal of management is prevention of osteoporosis by non-pharmacologic means.

Mrs. VG has type II diabetes mellitus. FRAX® score underestimates the fracture risk as it does not include diabetes mellitus, a risk factor for osteoporosis, falls, and fractures. The goal of management is treatment of low bone mass.

Mrs. BAC has Lewy Body Dementia and sustained several falls. In these patients the FRAX® score underestimates the fracture risk as it does not take into account the risk of falling. The goal of management is to treat the low bone mass and reduce the fall risk.

Figure 7.1 To Treat or Not to Treat Is a Clinical Decision.

Regardless of which medication is prescribed, lifestyle changes and secondary osteoporosis must be addressed so as to maximize the efficacy of the medication (see Chapter 6).

The efficacy of any medication is dependent on the patient's adherence, that is, compliance and persistence with the intake of the medication.[1] Adherence is low for osteoporosis and other chronic asymptomatic conditions (e.g., hypertension, hypercholesterolemia); therefore, patients must be motivated to start and to continue treatment. Noncompliance with the prescribed medication is associated with increased fracture risks.[2]

Osteoporosis is caused by an imbalance between bone resorption and bone formation resulting in more resorption than formation, leading to a reduced bone mass. Two general categories of therapeutic strategies are available: inhibit bone resorption (antiresorptives) or stimulate bone formation (osteoanabolics). Both strategies increase bone mass. As bone resorption and bone formation are coupled, the continuous inhibition of one may inhibit the other, and conversely the continuous stimulation of one may stimulate the other.

The main emphasis of this review focuses on fracture risk reduction and, to a lesser extent, changes in BMD and bone turnover markers (BTMs). Although very important, insightful, interesting, and attractive work is done on bone histomorphometry and structure, these issues will not be addressed in this text. The management of osteoporosis in men and glucocorticoid-induced osteoporosis are discussed in Chapters 11 and 14.

Bisphosphonates

All bisphosphonates share the same chemical structure: two phosphonic acid molecules joined to a carbon molecule and two side chains. Bisphosphonates reduce the bone resorptive activity of osteoclasts by selectively inhibiting intracellular farnesyl pyrophosphate synthase, the key regulatory enzyme in the mevalonic acid pathway. This prevents downstream protein prenylation, which in turn inhibits bone resorption and leads to osteoclast apoptosis.[3] The two side chains determine the affinity of the bisphosphonate to hydroxyapatite crystals in bone matrix and the degree to which bone resorption is inhibited. Differences in side chains account for differences in the pharmacological properties of various bisphosphonates.[4] The inhibitory activity is highest with zoledronic acid, followed by risedronate, ibandronate, and alendronate.[5] The binding affinity to hydroxyapatite crystals is highest with zoledronic acid, followed by alendronate, ibandronate and risedronate.[6]

Only 0.6 to 3%of the orally administered bisphosphonate is absorbed.[7] Any interference with absorption may further reduce bioavailability. Hence the importance of ensuring patients take the medication while fasting with about 6 ounces of water to ensure maximal dispersion, and to refrain from eating, drinking any fluid except water, or taking any other medication for 30 minutes in the case of alendronate or risedronate and 60 minutes for ibandronate. Because tap water, well water, spring water, or mineral water contains impurities or additives, some clinicians recommend bisphosphonates be taken with distilled water to ensure maximum absorption. The complexities of administering oral bisphosphonates discourages many patients from complying and persevering with their intake. Long-term adherence with oral bisphosphonate therapy is problematic.[8] Risedronate delayed release is an exception to other orally administered bisphosphonates: It is formulated in such a way that it can be taken immediately after breakfast. The active medication, risedronate, is enclosed in a pH-sensitive capsule that dissolves only in an alkaline medium, thus it passes unaffected through the stomach and dissolves in the small intestine. A chelating agent surrounds risedronate and when released binds to cations in the intestines, thus preventing them from interfering with risedronate absorption.

Alendronate

Alendronate is available for oral administration: 70 and 35 mg once a week, and 10 and 5 mg daily. The higher doses are for treatment, the lower doses for prevention. The daily dose is seldom used. Generic formulations are available.

Efficacy

Postmenopausal Osteoporosis

Fracture Intervention Trial (FIT)

Analysis of the Clinical fracture arm data shows that over a four-year period, alendronate reduced hip fractures by 56%, single morphometric vertebral fractures by 49%, multiple morphometric vertebral fractures by 60%, clinical fractures by 36%, and nonvertebral fractures by 35% compared with placebo. The increase in BMD compared with placebo was 6.6% in the lumbar vertebrae, 4.6% in the femoral neck, 6.8% in the trochanter, and 5% in the total hip. The study included 4,432 postmenopausal women between the ages of 54 and 81 years: 1,631 had densitometric evidence of osteoporosis (T-score −2.5 or less), whereas most of the others had osteopenia.[9]

Analysis of the Vertebral fracture arm data shows that over a 3-year period, alendronate reduced hip fractures by 51%, single morphometric vertebral fractures by 47%, multiple vertebral morphometric fractures by 90%, clinical vertebral fractures by 55%, wrist fractures by 48%, and all clinical fractures by 26% compared with placebo. The study included 2,027 women between the ages of 55 and 81 years, with a history of prior vertebral compression fracture and a mean T-score of −1.6.[10]

Pooled fracture intervention trial (clinical and vertebral fracture arms) analysis shows that compared with placebo, alendronate reduced clinical vertebral fractures (59%) by 12 months, hip fractures (63%) by 18 months, clinical nonvertebral fractures (26%) by 24 months, and wrist fractures (30%) by 30 months.[11]

Alendronate may be more effective in patients with a high rate of bone turnover. Compared with placebo, alendronate reduced the risk of nonvertebral fractures by 46% and 12% in patients with BTM in the highest and lowest tertiles, respectively.[12] The efficacy of alendronate is not reduced in older patients.[13]

Fosamax International Trial (FOSIT)

Over a 1-year period, alendronate reduced nonvertebral fractures by 47% and increased BMD by 4.9%, 2.4%, 3.6%, and 3.0% in the lumbar vertebrae, femoral neck, trochanter, and total hip, respectively compared with placebo. The study included 1,908 postmenopausal women, with lumbar spine T-score less than or equal to −2.0.[14]

- **Postmenopausal women with osteopenia:** Alendronate is effective at preventing bone loss in postmenopausal women with osteopenia. After a 6-year period, fractures occurred in 11.5%, 10.3%, and 8.9% of patients on placebo, alendronate 2.5 and 5 mg daily.[15]

- **Daily versus weekly dose:** Alendronate 10 mg once a day and 70 mg once a week have similar effects on changes in BMD and BTM.[16] Patients prefer the weekly dose and adherence is better.[17]

- **Long-term administration of alendronate:** In postmenopausal women with osteoporosis who have taken alendronate for 5 years, continuing it beyond 5 years further reduces the subsequent risk of nonvertebral fractures if at five years the T-score is −2.5 or lower. For those whose T-score after 5 years of treatment is higher than −2.0, continuing alendronate does not further reduce the risk of fractures.[18]

- **Alendronate and raloxifene:** In postmenopausal women 75 years old or younger with osteoporosis, alendronate increased lumbar vertebrae and femoral neck BMD to a larger extent than raloxifene, and the combination raloxifene+alendronate increased BMD to a larger extent than either medication at the lumbar vertebrae (raloxifene 2.1%, alendronate 4.3%, and raloxifene +alendronate 5.3%) and femoral neck (raloxifene 1.7%, alendronate 2.7%, and raloxifene+alendronate 3.7%). The effect of this combination on fracture risk is not known.[19]

Risedronate

Risedronate is available for oral administration 150 mg once a month or 35 mg once a week. The same dose is used for treatment and prevention. Two formulations are available: Conventional risedronate and risedronate delayed release. The former has to be taken as outlined for alendronate. The latter is taken immediately after breakfast.

Efficacy

- **Postmenopausal women with osteoporosis:**
  - Hip Intervention Program (HIP). Over a 3-year period compared with placebo, risedronate reduced the risk of hip fractures by 60% in subjects who had a vertebral compression fracture before inclusion in the study, and 40% in those who did not have such fractures. Hip fracture risk was reduced by 20% in those aged 80 years and older. The study included 5,445 postmenopausal women with osteoporosis between the ages of 70 and 79 years and 3,886 women aged 80 years or older. Subjects between the ages of 70 and 79 years were recruited based on a T-score of −4.0 or lower or a T-score of −3.0 or lower if, in addition, they had evidence of at least one nonskeletal risk factor for hip fracture. Those aged 80 years and older were included based on densitometric evidence or nonskeletal risk factors for fractures. Therefore, it is possible that some in this older group did not have osteoporosis.[20]
  - Vertebral Efficacy with Risedronate Therapy (VERT) Study. Over a 3-year period compared with placebo, patients on risedronate had 41% fewer

new vertebral fractures. Significant reductions in fracture risk (62%) were observed after 1 year of treatment with risedronate compared with placebo.[21] Similarly, compared with placebo, the BMD increased significantly at the lumbar vertebrae (5.4% vs. 1.1%), femoral neck (1.6% vs. −1.2%), and trochanter (3.3% vs. −0.7%). This study included 2,458 and 1,116 ambulatory postmenopausal women younger than 85 years with at least one vertebral fracture in the North American and Multinational groups, respectively.[22]

- Risedronate may be more effective in patients with a high rate of bone turnover: The number of patients needed to treat to prevent one vertebral compression fracture at 12 months is 15 for those with high levels of BTMs compared with 25 for those with low BTMs levels.[23]
- Risedronate is effective in patients aged 80 years and older: Over a 1-year period compared with placebo, the risk of new vertebral fractures was 81% lower in patients on risedronate. In this age group the number of women needed to treat for 1 year to prevent one vertebral fracture was 12.[24]

- *Postmenopausal women with osteopenia:* In a post hoc analysis of four clinical trials, risedronate reduced the risk of fragility fractures by 73% in patients with osteopenia.[25]
- *Post hip fracture:* When administered to patients post hip fracture, the risk of subsequent contralateral hip fracture was 4.3% in the risedronate group and 13.1% in the control group. The 36-month prospective study included 529 patients: 173 on risedronate and 356 untreated controls.[26]
- *Hip fracture prevention in patients with neurologic diseases:* Risedronate reduced the risk of hip fractures in patients who have sustained strokes, or have Parkinson's or Alzheimer's disease.[27–30]
- *Patients on aromatase inhibitors:* Risedronate prevents bone loss in oncology patients treated with aromatase inhibitors.[31,32]
- *Prevention of periprosthetic bone resorption:* Risedronate reduces periprosthetic bone resorption around uncemented femoral stems.[33]

Monthly versus Weekly versus Daily Dose

The weekly (35 mg) and monthly (150 mg) doses were as effective as the daily dose (5 mg) at increasing BMD.[34] All doses were well tolerated, but more patients in the monthly group experienced an acute phase reaction than in the daily group: 1.4% versus 0.2%.

Delayed-Release Formulation

The delayed-release formulation administered after breakfast has the same effect on BTMs and BMD as risedronate 5 mg taken 30 minutes before breakfast. This study included 767 postmenopausal women with osteoporosis. The delayed release formulation simplifies the dosing regimen.[35]

Discontinuing Risedronate

Discontinuing risedronate after it had been administered for 2 to 7 years leads to a gradual increase in BTMs and a decrease in BMD in the total hip and femoral trochanter.[36]

Risedronate versus Alendronate: Retrospective Observational Study

A retrospective observational cohort study on postmenopausal women aged 65 years and older identified 12,215 who had been on risedronate and 21,615 on alendronate for 1 year. The risks of hip and nonvertebral fractures were reduced by 43% and 18% in the risedronate and alendronate cohorts, respectively.[37]

Ibandronate

Ibandronate is available as tablets (150 mg monthly) or intravenous formulation 3 mg/3 mL every 3 months.

Efficacy

- *Postmenopausal osteoporosis:* Over a 3-year period compared with placebo, ibandronate reduced the risk of new vertebral fractures by 62% in postmenopausal women with a lumbar spine T-score of –2.0 or lower. The BMD of the lumbar spine was increased by 6.5% versus 1.3% in the placebo group. The study included 2,946 postmenopausal women. Although in the entire group there were no differences in the rate of nonvertebral fractures, a post hoc analysis of patients with femoral neck T-scores lower than –3.0 showed that in this subgroup ibandronate reduced the risk of nonvertebral fractures by 69%. It was well tolerated.[38]

- *Osteopenia in postmenopausal women:* Oral formulation: In postmenopausal women with osteopenia, ibandronate 2.5 mg daily increased the BMD of the lumbar vertebrae by 3.1% over a 2-year period compared with placebo (1.8%). BTMs were decreased. The study included 653 postmenopausal women with osteopenia.[39]

- *Intravenous formulation*: Compared with placebo, ibandronate administered intravenously every 3 months for 1 year to 629 postmenopausal women with osteopenia increased the BMD of the lumbar vertebrae and hip in a dose-dependent fashion: 2.5%, 1.8%, and 1% for the 2 mg, 1 mg, and 0.5 mg doses, respectively. Similarly decreases in BTMs were dose dependent.[40]

30 versus 60 Minutes Before Breakfast

Administering ibandronate 30 minutes rather than 60 minutes before breakfast for 48 weeks induced smaller increases in the BMD of the lumbar vertebrae (3.07% vs. 4.95), trochanter (3.04% vs. 4.36%), femoral neck (1.82 vs. 2.19%), and total hip (2.35% vs. 3.21%). Similarly, suppression of BTMs was less in the 30- than 60-minute group: C-telopeptide (CTX) (–48.5% vs. –61.8%) and osteocalcin (–34.8% vs. 43.8%). These findings emphasize the importance of a 60-minute fast after taking ibandronate.[41]

Reduced Oral Dosing Frequency/Intravenous Route: Noninferiority Studies

The oral 1- and 3-month intravenous doses are not inferior to the daily oral dose.[42,43]

Patients' Preferences

Patients prefer monthly to weekly dosage.[44]

Zoledronic Acid

Zoledronic acid (ZOL), 5 mg in a 100 mL ready-to-infuse intravenously solution, is available for the treatment (once a year) and prevention (once every other year) of osteoporosis. The intravenous administration bypasses the gastrointestinal (GI) tract, is not associated with upper GI adverse effects, and improves adherence.[45] Patients prefer it to weekly oral bisphosphonates.[46] It is contraindicated in patients who have a creatinine clearance less than 35 mL/minute, hypocalcemia, are hypersensitive to ZOL or any bisphosphonate, are pregnant or nursing mothers, or are on other forms of ZOL.

Efficacy

- **Postmenopausal osteoporosis:** Health Outcomes and Reduced Incidence with Zoledronic Acid Once Yearly-Pivotal Fracture Trial (HORIZON-PFT). Over a 3-year period compared with placebo, ZOL reduced hip fractures by 41%, new morphometric vertebral fractures by 70%, and nonvertebral fractures by 25%. It increased the BMD by 6% in the total hip, 5.1% in the femoral neck, and 6.7% in the lumbar vertebrae. At the end of 12 months there were significant decreases in BTMs. The study included 7,765 postmenopausal women between the ages of 65 and 89 years with a T-score of −2.5 or lower at the femoral neck or a T-score of −1.5 and lower if they also had radiologic evidence of either one moderate or two mild vertebral compression fractures. The overall incidence of adverse events was similar in ZOL and placebo groups, except for the acute phase reaction which was higher in ZOL group, but decreased with subsequent infusions.[47] A 3-year extension of this study when patients were randomly allocated to continue with ZOL or go on placebo, showed that there were fewer morphologic fractures in ZOL than placebo group: 14 versus 30 fractures.[48] ZOL is equally effective in older and younger patients.[49]
- **Post fragility hip fractures:** HORIZON-Recurrent Fracture Trial (HORIZON-RFT). In patients who have sustained a fragility hip fracture within the previous 90 days, ZOL compared with placebo reduced the risk of subsequent clinical fractures by 35% and overall mortality by 28%. This study included 2,127 patients: 1,619 women and 508 men; mean ages were 74.6 ± 9.86 years and 74.4 ± 9.48 years in placebo and ZOL groups, respectively.[50] A subsequent time interval analysis showed that the administration of ZOL 2 or more weeks after surgical repair was associated with significant reductions in clinical fractures as well as increases in hip BMD.[51]
- **Postmenopausal women with osteopenia:** Over a 2-year period compared with placebo, postmenopausal women receiving ZOL had a 5.18% increase in the BMD of the lumbar vertebrae and decreases in BTMs. This study was conducted on 581 women 45 years or older with a T-score between −1.0 and −2.5.[52]

Other Conditions Associated with Bone Demineralization

- **Cancer-related osteoporosis:** ZOL is effective in the management of osteoporosis in oncology patients on aromatase inhibitors or androgen deprivation therapy.[53] It is also useful in patients with bone metastases.[54]

When administered in conjunction with adjuvant endocrine therapy, ZOL improves the disease-free survival of premenopausal women with endocrine-responsive breast cancer.[55]

- **Bone demineralization following strokes:** ZOL prevented significant bone loss at the hip in 27 patients with hemiplegia.[56]
- **Patients with human immunodeficiency virus (HIV) and low bone mass:** ZOL is beneficial to HIV patients with a low bone mass.[57]

Switching Alendronate to Zoledronic Acid Therapy

A 5 mg intravenous infusion of ZOL to patients who had been on alendronate 70 mg weekly for at least 1 year maintained the lumbar vertebrae BMD, and 78.7% of the patients preferred the once-a-year infusion to the weekly alendronate tablets.[46]

Adverse Drug Effects of Bisphosphonates

Gastrointestinal Adverse Drug Effects

Phosphonic acid is an irritant to the GI mucosa and may induce heartburn, dyspepsia, chest pain, abdominal pain, or cramps. To minimize these adverse effects, patients should not engage in activities that increase the risk of gastroesophageal reflux, including lying down, semireclining in a lounger, doing housework, or jogging for 30 to 60 minutes after taking the tablet. Consuming a high-fiber meal coats the bisphosphonate particles that have not been absorbed (at least 97% of the dose), thus reducing the potential of irritating the GI mucosa. There are conflicting data on the relationship between oral bisphosphonates and esophageal cancer.[58]

Musculoskeletal Pain

Occasionally patients complain of severe, sometimes incapacitating, musculoskeletal pain in the lower back, pelvis, hips, thighs, knees, and ribs after taking bisphosphonates.[59] Although often spontaneously relieved, the pain sometimes lingers, even after discontinuing the bisphosphonate. As the pain occurs more frequently in patients with low vitamin D levels and secondary hyperparathyroidism, it is possible that the increased rate of bone turnover leads to a higher concentration of the bisphosphonate in the bone microenvironment, which increases the production of interleukin-6 and other proinflammatory cytokines, thus triggering an inflammatory response.[60] Causality between bisphosphonate treatment and musculoskeletal pain has not been established. Other causes of acute musculoskeletal pains include synovitis,[61] acute polyarthritis, myalgia,[62] and osteoarthritis flare-up.[63]

Arrhythmias and Atrial Fibrillation

In the HORIZON-PFT study, arrhythmias occurred in 6.9% of patients receiving ZOL and 5.3% of those on placebo. Serious atrial fibrillation occurred in 1.3% of patients on ZOL and 0.5% of those on placebo.[64] In 47 of the 50 patients who developed atrial fibrillation, the onset of the arrhythmia was more than 30 days after the intravenous infusion, reducing the likelihood of being related to acute hypocalcemia, electrolyte, or other homeostatic changes. Although earlier clinical trials on bisphosphonates were not designed to assess such events, causality between bisphosphonate treatment and atrial fibrillation has not been established. A meta-analysis of studies comparing alendronate with placebo did not substantiate an increased risk of atrial fibrillation.[65]

Acute Phase Reaction

Acute phase reaction is the main adverse effect of intravenously administered bisphosphonates. Patients experience a variety of symptoms, including low-grade temperature, generalized aches and pains, fatigue, malaise, and lethargy. It tends to occur within 24 to 36 hours of the infusion and is usually self-limited, most symptoms subsiding spontaneously within 3 to 4 days. The intensity of the symptoms decreases with subsequent infusions. It affects about 18% of bisphosphonate-naïve patients, but only 9% of patients previously exposed to bisphosphonates. Its incidence and severity can be reduced by acetaminophen or ibuprofen.[66] The acute phase reaction is occasionally seen in patients administered the first monthly or weekly dose of oral bisphosphonates.

Nephrotoxicity

A few (1.3%) patients administered ZOL had a transient increase in serum creatinine of more than 0.5 mg/dL compared with 0.4% of patients administered placebo. Within 30 days the serum creatinine levels returned to baseline in about 85% of the subjects.[67] Over a 6-year period, annual infusions of ZOL did not result in any significant renal impairment.[48] The present evidence suggests that ibandronate does not induce nephrotoxicity even in patients with abnormal baseline renal functions.[68]

Hypocalcemia

By reducing the rate of bone resorption, bisphosphonates, especially intravenously administered ones, may reduce the mobilization of calcium from bones to blood and lead to transient hypocalcemia. Patients with hypovitaminosis D, renal impairment, or hypoparathyroidism may not be able to rapidly compensate for the drop in serum calcium level. In the HORIZON-PFT study 0.2% of patients receiving ZOL exhibited a mild (<1.87 mmol/L) decrease in the serum calcium level. Although in most instances asymptomatic, hypocalcemia may present with numbness and tingling sensations around the mouth. Muscle spasms or cramps are rarely seen. Patients should be normocalcemic before administering intravenous bisphosphonates.[69]

Ocular Adverse Effects

Ocular adverse effects are rare, idiosyncratic, usually benign complications of bisphosphonate therapy except for uveitis and scleritis, which necessitate prompt medical attention.[70] Patients present with ocular pain, photophobia, and/or impaired vision. Nonspecific conjunctivitis is usually self-limiting. Ocular complications may occur weeks, months, or even years after the initiation of bisphosphonate therapy.[71]

Skin Reactions

Skin reactions including rash, pruritus, Stevens-Johnson syndrome, and toxic epidermal necrolysis have been reported in patients on bisphosphonates.[72]

Medication	Study Acronym	Number of Patients Included	Fracture Risk Reduction		Postmenopausal Osteoporosis		Men	References Chapter	
			Hip	Vertebral	Treatment	Prevention		7	8
Bisphosphonates									
Alendronate	FIT-CFA ; FIT-VFA FOSIT	4,432; 2,027; 1,908	Yes	Yes	Yes	Yes	Yes	9, 10, 14	
Ibandronate	BONE	2,946	No*	Yes	Yes	Yes	No	38	
Risedronate	HIP; VERT(NA) VERT(MN)	5,445; 2,458; 1,116	Yes	Yes	Yes	Yes	Yes	20, 21, 22	
Zoledronic acid	HORIZON-PFT HORIZON-RFT	7,765 2,127	Yes	Yes	Yes	Yes	Yes	47, 48, 51	
Calcitonin	PROOF	1,255	No*	Yes	Yes	No	No		50
Denosumab	FREEDOM	7,868	Yes	Yes	No	No	Yes		34, 37
Raloxifene	MORE	7,705	No*	Yes	Yes	Yes	Yes		59
Teriparatide	FPT; EFOS	1,637; 1,649	**	Yes	Yes	No	Yes	9, 11	

* The lack of demonstrable effect may be due to studies not being powered to this end-point.

** The pivotal study had to be prematurely terminated to evaluate the osteosarcoma risk.

Figure 7.2 Major Pivotal Studies with Fractures as Endpoints.

Rare Complications Possibly Associated with Long-Term Bisphosphonate Therapy

Atypical femoral shaft fractures and osteonecrosis of the jaw are discussed in Chapters 16 and 17 (Fig. 7.2).

References

1. Ross S, Samuels E, Gairy K, et al. A meta-analysis of osteoporotic fracture risk with medication nonadherence. Value Health. 2011;14(4):571–81.

2. Landfeldt E, Ström O, Robbins S, et al. Adherence to treatment of primary osteoporosis and its association to fractures—the Swedish Adherence Register Analysis (SARA). Osteoporos Int. 2012;23(2):433–43.

3. Kavanagh KL, Guo K, Dunford JE, et al. The molecular mechanism of nitrogen-containing bisphosphonates as antiosteoporosis drugs. Proc Natl Acad Sci U S A. 2006;103(20):7829–34.

4. Rizzoli R. Bisphosphonates for post-menopausal osteoporosis: are they all the same? QJM 2011;104(4):281–300.

5. Russell RGG. Determinants of structure-function relationships among bisphosphonates. Bone. 2007;40(5, supplement 2):S21–S25.

6. Nancollas GH, Tang R, Phipps RJ, et al. Novel insights into actions of bisphosphonates on bone: differences in interactions with hydroxyapatite. Bone. 2006;38(5):617–27.

7. Chapurlat RD, Delmas PD. Drug insight: Bisphosphonates for postmenopausal osteoporosis. Nat Clin Pract Endocrinol Metab. 2006;2(4):211–19.

8. Reginster JY, Rabenda V. Patient preference in the management of postmenopausal osteoporosis with bisphosphonates. Clin Interv Aging 2006;1:415–23.

9. Cummings SR, Black DM, Thompson DE, et al. Effect of alendronate on risk of fracture in women with low bone density but without vertebral fractures: results from the Fracture Intervention Trial. JAMA. 1998;280(24):2077–82.

10. Black DM, Cummings SR, Karpf DB, et al. Randomised trial of effect of alendronate on risk of fracture in women with existing vertebral fractures. Fracture Intervention Trial Research Group. Lancet. 1996;348(9041):1535–41.

11. Black DM, Thompson DE, Bauer DC, et al. Fracture risk reduction with alendronate in women with osteoporosis: the Fracture Intervention Trial. FIT Research Group. J Clin Endocrinol Metab. 2000;85(11):4118–24.

12. Bauer DC, Garnero P, Hochberg MC, et al. Pretreatment levels of bone turnover and the antifracture efficacy of alendronate: the fracture intervention trial. J Bone Miner Res. 2006;21(2):292–99.

13. Hochberg MC, Thompson DE, Black DM, et al. Effect of alendronate on the age-specific incidence of symptomatic osteoporotic fractures. J Bone Miner Res. 2005;20(6):971–76.

14. Pols HA, Felsenberg D, Hanley DA, et al. Multinational, placebo-controlled, randomized trial of the effects of alendronate on bone density and fracture risk in postmenopausal women with low bone mass: results of the FOSIT study. Fosamax International Trial Study Group. Osteoporos Int. 1999;9(5):461–68.

15. McClung MR, Wasnich RD, Hosking DJ, et al. Prevention of postmenopausal bone loss: six-year results from the Early Postmenopausal Intervention Cohort Study. J Clin Endocrinol Metab. 2004;89(10):4879–85.

16. Schnitzer T, Bone HG, Crepaldi G, et al. Therapeutic equivalence of alendronate 70 mg once-weekly and alendronate 10 mg daily in the treatment of osteoporosis. Alendronate Once-Weekly Study Group. Aging (Milano). 2000;12(1):1–12.

17. McCombs JS, Thiebaud P, McLaughlin-Miley C, et al. Compliance with drug therapies for the treatment and prevention of osteoporosis. Maturitas. 2004;48(3):271–87.

18. Schwartz AV, Bauer DC, Cummings SR, et al. Efficacy of continued alendronate for fractures in women with and without prevalent vertebral fracture: the FLEX trial. J Bone Miner Res. 2010;25(5):976–82.

19. Johnell O, Scheele WH, Lu Y, et al. Additive effects of raloxifene and alendronate on bone density and biochemical markers of bone remodeling in postmenopausal women with osteoporosis. Clin Endocrinol Metab. 2002;87(3):985–92.

20. McClung MR, Geusens P, Miller PD, et al. Effect of risedronate on the risk of hip fracture in elderly women. Hip Intervention Program Study Group. N Engl J Med. 2001;344(5):333–40.

21. Watts NB, Josse RG, Hamdy RC, et al. Risedronate prevents new vertebral fractures in postmenopausal women at high risk. J Clin Endocrinol Metab. 2003;88(2):542–49.

22. Harris ST, Watts NB, Genant HK, et al. Effects of risedronate treatment on vertebral and nonvertebral fractures in women with postmenopausal osteoporosis: a randomized controlled trial. Vertebral Efficacy With Risedronate Therapy (VERT) Study Group. JAMA. 1999;282(14):1344–52.

23. Seibel MJ, Naganathan V, Barton I, et al. Relationship between pretreatment bone resorption and vertebral fracture incidence in postmenopausal osteoporotic women treated with risedronate. J Bone Miner Res. 2004;19(2):323–29.

24. Boonen S, McClung MR, Eastell R, et al. Safety and efficacy of risedronate in reducing fracture risk in osteoporotic women aged 80 and older: implications for the use of anti-resorptive agents in the old and oldest old. J Am Geriatr Soc. 2004;52(11):1832–39.

25. Siris ES, Simon JA, Barton IP, et al. Effects of risedronate on fracture risk in postmenopausal women with osteopenia. Osteoporos Int. 2008;19(5):681–86.

26. Osaki M, Tatsuki K, Hashikawa T, et al. Beneficial effect of risedronate for preventing recurrent hip fracture in the elderly Japanese women. Osteoporos Int. 2012;23(2):695–703.

27. Sato Y, Iwamoto J, Kanoko T, et al. Risedronate sodium therapy for prevention of hip fracture in men 65 years or older after stroke. Arch Intern Med. 2005;165(15):1743–48.

28. Sato Y, Iwamoto J, Kanoko T, et al. Risedronate therapy for prevention of hip fracture after stroke in elderly women. Neurology 2005;64:811–16.

29. Sato Y, Honda Y, Iwamoto J. Risedronate and ergocalciferol prevent hip fracture in elderly men with Parkinson disease. Neurology. 2007;68(12):911–15.

30. Sato Y, Kanoko T, Satoh K, et al. The prevention of hip fracture with risedronate and ergocalciferol plus calcium supplementation in elderly women with Alzheimer disease: a randomized controlled trial. Arch Intern Med. 2005;165(15):1737–42.

31. Van Poznak C, Hannon RA, Mackey JR, et al. Prevention of aromatase inhibitor-induced bone loss using risedronate: the SABRE trial. J Clin Oncol. 2010;28(6):967–75.

32. Sergi G, Pintore G, Falci C, et al. Preventive effect of risedronate on bone loss and frailty fractures in elderly women treated with anastrozole for early breast cancer. J Bone Miner Metab. 2011 Dec 13. [Epub ahead of print]

33. Sköldenberg OG, Salemyr MO, Bodén HS, et al. The effect of weekly risedronate on periprosthetic bone resorption following total hip arthroplasty: a randomized, double-blind, placebo-controlled trial. J Bone Joint Surg Am. 2011;93(20):1857–64.

34. Delmas PD, McClung MR, Zanchetta JR, et al. Efficacy and safety of risedronate 150 mg once a month in the treatment of postmenopausal osteoporosis. Bone. 2008;42(1):36–42.

35. McClung MR, Miller PD, Brown JP, et al. Efficacy and safety of a novel delayed-release risedronate 35 mg once-a-week tablet. Osteoporos Int. 2012;23(1):267–76.

36. Eastell R, Hannon RA, Wenderoth D, et al. Effect of stopping risedronate after long-term treatment on bone turnover. J Clin Endocrinol Metab. 2011;96(11):3367–73.

37. Silverman SL, Watts NB, Delmas PD, et al. Effectiveness of bisphosphonates on nonvertebral and hip fractures in the first year of therapy: the risedronate and alendronate (REAL) cohort study. Osteoporos Int. 2007;18(1):25–34.

38. Chesnut III CH, Skag A, Christiansen C, et al. Effects of oral ibandronate administered daily or intermittently on fracture risk in postmenopausal osteoporosis. J Bone Miner Res. 2004;19(8):1241–49.

39. McClung MR, Wasnich RD, Recker R, et al. Oral daily ibandronate prevents bone loss in early postmenopausal women without osteoporosis. J Bone Miner Res. 2004;19(1):11–18.

40. Stakkestad JA, Benevolenskaya LI, Stepan JJ, et al. Intravenous ibandronate injections given every three months: a new treatment option to prevent bone loss in postmenopausal women. Ann Rheum Dis. 2003;62(10):969–75.

41. Tankó LB, McClung MR, Schimmer RC, et al. The efficacy of 48-week oral ibandronate treatment in postmenopausal osteoporosis when taken 30 versus 60 minutes before breakfast. Bone. 2003;32(4):421–26.

42. Stakkestad JA, Lakatos P, Lorenc R, et al. Monthly oral ibandronate is effective and well tolerated after 3 years: the MOBILE long-term extension. Clin Rheumatol. 2008;27(8):955–60.

43. Eisman JA, Civitelli R, Adami S, et al. Efficacy and tolerability of intravenous ibandronate injections in postmenopausal osteoporosis: 2-year results from the DIVA study. J Rheumatol. 2008;35(3):488–97.

44. Cotté FE, Fardellone P, Mercier F, et al. Adherence to monthly and weekly oral bisphosphonates in women with osteoporosis. Osteoporos Int. 2010;21(1):145–55.

45. Hamdy RC. Zoledronic acid: clinical utility and patient considerations in osteoporosis and low bone mass. Drug Des Devel Ther. 2010;4:321–35.

46. McClung M, Recker R, Miller P, et al. Intravenous zoledronic acid 5 mg in the treatment of postmenopausal women with low bone density previously treated with alendronate. Bone. 2007;41(1):122–28.

47. Black DM, Delmas PD, Eastell R, et al. Once-yearly zoledronic acid for treatment of postmenopausal osteoporosis. N Engl J Med. 2007;356(18):1809–22.

48. Black DM, Reid IR, Boonen S, et al. The effect of 3 versus 6 years of zoledronic acid treatment of osteoporosis: a randomized extension to the HORIZON-Pivotal Fracture Trial (PFT). J Bone Miner Res 2012;27:243–54.

49. Boonen S, Black DM, Colón-Emeric CS, et al. Efficacy and safety of a once-yearly intravenous zoledronic acid 5 mg for fracture prevention in elderly postmenopausal women with osteoporosis aged 75 and older. J Am Geriatr Soc. 2010;58(2):292–99.

50. Lyles KW, Colón-Emeric CS, Magaziner JS, et al. Zoledronic acid and clinical fractures and mortality after hip fracture. N Engl J Med 2007;357:1799–1809.

51. Eriksen EF, Lyles KW, Colón-Emeric CS, et al. Antifracture efficacy and reduction of mortality in relation to timing of the first dose of zoledronic acid after hip fracture. J Bone Miner Res. 2009;24(7):1308–13.

52. McClung M, Miller P, Recknor C, et al. Zoledronic acid for the prevention of bone loss in postmenopausal women with low bone mass: a randomized controlled trial. Obstet Gynecol. 2009;114(5):999–1007.

53. Hines SL, Sloan JA, Atherton PJ, et al. Zoledronic acid for treatment of osteopenia and osteoporosis in women with primary breast cancer undergoing adjuvant aromatase inhibitor therapy. Breast. 2010;19(2):92–96.

54. Polascik TJ, Mouraviev V. Zoledronic acid in the management of metastatic bone disease. Therap Clin Risk Manag 2008;4:261–68.

55. Gnant M, Mlineritsch B, Schippinger W, et al. Endocrine therapy plus zoledronic acid in premenopausal breast cancer. N Engl J Med. 2009;360(7):679–91.

56. Poole KE, Loveridge N, Rose CM, et al. A single infusion of zoledronate prevents bone loss after stroke. Stroke. 2007;38(5):1519–25.

57. Huang J, Meixner L, Fernandez S, et al. A double-blinded, randomized controlled trial of zoledronate therapy for HIV-associated osteopenia and osteoporosis. AIDS. 2009;23(1):51–57.

58. Haber SL, McNatty D. An evaluation of the use of oral bisphosphonates and risk of esophageal cancer. Ann Pharmacother. 2012;46(3):419–23.

59. Wysowski DK, Chang JT. Alendronate and risedronate: reports of severe bone, joint, and muscle pain. Arch Intern Med. 2005;165(3):346–47.

60. de Torrenté de la Jara G, Pécoud A, Favrat B. Musculoskeletal pain in female asylum seekers and hypovitaminosis D3. BMJ. 2004;329(7458):156–57.

61. Gwynne Jones DP, Savage RL, Highton J. Alendronate-induced synovitis. J Rheumatol. 2008;35(3):537–38.

62. Gerster JH. Acute polyarthritis related to once-weekly alendronate in a woman with osteoporosis. J Rheumatol. 2004;31(4):829–30.

63. Werner de Castro GR, Neves FS, de Magalhães Souza Fialho SC, et al. Flare-up of hand osteoarthritis caused by zoledronic acid infusion. Osteoporos Int. 2010;21(9):1617–19.

64. Pazianas M, Compston J, Huang CL. Atrial fibrillation and bisphosphonate therapy. J Bone Miner Res. 2010;25(1):2–10.

65. Barrett-Connor E, Swern AS, Hustad CM, et al. Alendronate and atrial fibrillation: a meta-analysis of randomized placebo-controlled clinical trials. Osteoporos Int. 2012;23(1):233–45.

66. Wark JD, Bensen W, Recknor C, et al. Treatment with acetaminophen/paracetamol or ibuprofen alleviates post-dose symptoms related to intravenous infusion with zoledronic acid 5 mg. Osteoporos Int. 2012;23(2):503–12.

67. Boonen S, Sellmeyer DE, Lippuner K, et al. Renal safety of annual zoledronic acid infusions in osteoporotic postmenopausal women. Kidney Int. 2008 Sep;74(5):641–48.

68. Perazella MA, Markowitz GS. Bisphosphonate nephrotoxicity. Kidney Int. 2008;74(11):1385–93.

69. Lambrinoudaki I, Vlachou S, Galapi F, et al. Once-yearly zoledronic acid in the prevention of osteoporotic bone fractures in postmenopausal women. Clin Interv Aging. 2008;3(3):445–51.

70. Papapetrou PD. Bisphosphonate-associated adverse events. Hormones (Athens). 2009;8(2):96–110.

71. Procianoy F, Procianoy E. Orbital inflammatory disease secondary to a single-dose administration of zoledronic acid for treatment of postmenopausal osteoporosis. Osteoporos Int. 2010;21(6):1057–58.

72. Abrahamsen B. Adverse effects of bisphosphonates. Calcif Tissue Int. 2010;86(6):421–35.

Chapter 8

Pharmacologic Management of Osteoporosis, Part 2

Teriparatide

Teriparatide (recombinant human parathyroid hormone 1–34) is an osteoanabolic agent available as 20 mcg daily subcutaneous injections. It stimulates bone formation, increases bone turnover, increases bone mineral density (BMD), and reduces fracture risk. Its administration induces initial large increases in bone turnover markers (BTMs) and BMD during the first 6 to 12 months of therapy; thereafter the effect gradually wanes. Neither the readministration of teriparatide after a hiatus of 1 year,[1] nor the gradual escalation of the administered dose[2] recaptures the marked initial increases in BMD and BTMs. The maximum duration of therapy with teriparatide in the United States has been set at 24 months in a lifetime. Unless an antiresorptive agent is administered, discontinuation of teriparatide is associated with loss of BMD.[3–5] Patient compliance and persistence with daily subcutaneous injections is good: 89% at 6 months and 82% at 18 months.[6] The high cost of teriparatide is a factor impacting initiation and persistence with treatment.[7] Alternate delivery methods have been studied; a micro-needle patch delivery system seems promising.[8]

Efficacy

- *Postmenopausal women with osteoporosis:*
  - Fracture Prevention Trial (FPT). Compared with placebo, patients administered teriparatide (20 and 40 mcg) daily sc injections sustained fewer new vertebral fractures: 14% in the placebo group, and 5% and 4% in the 20 and 40 mcg teriparatide groups, respectively. New nonvertebral fractures were also reduced: 6% in the placebo group and 3% in each of the teriparatide groups. Compared with placebo, both doses increased BMD in the lumbar vertebrae, 9% and 13%; femoral neck, 3% and 6%; and total body, 2% and 4%, respectively. This study included 1,637 postmenopausal women with at least one moderate or two mild atraumatic vertebral compression fractures, or if they had fewer than two vertebral fractures, a T-score of −1.0 or lower in the hip or lumbar vertebrae. Teriparatide was well tolerated. The study was terminated prematurely to evaluate the clinical relevance of osteosarcomas developing in Fischer-344 rats during a toxicology study.[9]
  - The antifracture effect of teriparatide persists after the medication is stopped. A follow-up study included 1,071 women: 353, 373, and 345 had been on placebo, 20 and 40 mcg teriparatide, respectively. By the end of

18-month follow-up, 52%, 44%, and 46% of the subjects who had been in the placebo, 20 and 40 mcg groups, respectively, reported using a medication for osteoporosis. In the placebo group 19% of the subjects sustained one or more vertebral fractures compared with 11.3% and 10.4% of those who had been on the 20 and 40 mcg doses. Fewer patients complained of back pain if they had been on teriparatide than placebo: 19.8%, 14.0%, and 12.9% for placebo, 20 and 40 mcg teriparatide groups, respectively.[10] An extension of this study for another 18 months confirmed the sustained fracture protection effect.[11]

- The European Forsteo Observational Study (EFOS) enrolled 1,649 post-menopausal women about to start teriparatide therapy. Patients were followed during the 18-month teriparatide treatment period and for 18 months thereafter; 73.7% of the patients had been treated with bisphosphonates before enrolling in the study and 70.7% received medication for osteoporosis during the 18-month post-teriparatide period. The number of fractures/10,000 patient years steadily decreased from a highest level (1,119) in the first 6 months of teriparatide therapy to 815 and 645 in the following 6-month periods. The decrease continued after teriparatide therapy was discontinued: 606, 387, and 327 fractures/10,000 patient years for each 6-month period. The decrease in back pain was maintained after discontinuation of teriparatide therapy. The most common adverse events during teriparatide therapy were nausea (5.4%) and headaches (4.3%).[12]

- *Osteoporosis in older people:* The efficacy of teriparatide is not reduced in older patients. In addition to increased BMD and reduced fracture risk, consumption of nonsteroidal anti-inflammatory medications was reduced by about 80% and improvement was noted in the Quality-of-Life Questionnaire (European Foundation for Osteoporosis). The 24-month study included 141 older women (mean age 73.4 ± 5.8 years) with severe osteoporosis who had sustained an average of 3 ± 0.85 fragility fractures and whose mean T-scores in the lumbar vertebrae and femoral neck were −3.15 ± 0.39 and −2.5 ± 0.28, respectively. Teriparatide was administered for 18 months and the subjects were followed up for another 6 months. All had been on antiresorptives for at least 1 year before inclusion in the study.[13]

- *Back pain:* Studies have documented the beneficial effects of teriparatide on back pain and quality of life parameters.[12]

- *Other potential uses:* Given the osteoanabolic effect of teriparatide, it is sometimes used off-label in a number of conditions, including stress fractures,[14] osteonecrosis of the jaw (see Chapter 17), aseptic loosening of the hip prosthesis following hemiarthroplasty,[15] severe chronic periodontitis,[16] pregnancy-associated severe osteoporosis,[17] severe refractory hypocalcemia post renal transplant,[18] and post-parathyroidectomy for primary hyperparathyroidism in patients at risk of sustaining fractures.[19]

Preventing Loss of BMD After Discontinuing Teriparatide

To maintain the gains in BMD induced by teriparatide, an antiresorptive agent should be prescribed when teriparatide is discontinued.[3,20] Starting bisphosphonate therapy immediately on discontinuing teriparatide is associated with further increases in lumbar spine BMD.[21] The administration of raloxifene after discontinuing teriparatide attenuates bone loss, but does not increase bone mass.[22]

The simultaneous administration of teriparatide and antiresorptive therapy does not provide an advantage over monotherapy,[3,23,24] although increases in BMD may be more pronounced in the first 6 months.[25] Raloxifene may enhance the osteoanabolic effect of teriparatide.[26]

Switching Therapy to Teriparatide

Whereas treatment with raloxifene before teriparatide therapy does not interfere with the effects of teriparatide on BMD and BTMs, previous treatment with alendronate and, to a lesser extent, risedronate, may blunt the response to teriparatide.[27]

Osteosarcoma

A dose- and duration-dependent increased incidence of osteosarcoma, osteoblastoma, and osteoma in Fisher-344 rats was observed in a toxicology study[28] when rats were administered teriparatide in doses 3, 20, and 60 times higher than the exposure of humans receiving daily subcutaneous 20 mcg doses. The incidence of bone tumors was not increased in ovariectomized female monkeys administered teriparatide in doses approximately six times those administered to humans for 18 months and followed up for 3 years.[28]

The clinical relevance of the increased osteosarcoma incidence among the Fischer-344 rats is uncertain. Notwithstanding, teriparatide should not be administered to children and young adults with open epiphyses, patients with skeletal malignancies, bone metastases, hyperparathyroidism, hypercalcemia, Paget's disease of bone, unexplained elevated serum alkaline phosphatase levels, patients who have received external beam or implant radiation involving the skeleton, or those who have metabolic bone diseases other than osteoporosis.

Denosumab

Denosumab is available as a 60 mg solution administered sc at 6-month intervals for the treatment of osteoporosis. The antiresorptive activity of denosumab is mediated through the inhibition of osteoclast formation and activation. Its route of administration appeals to many patients, and many prefer it to weekly tablets.[29]Denosumab is a fully human monoclonal immunoglobulin G2 antibody with high affinity and specificity to receptor activator of nuclear factor-kappa-B ligand (RANKL).[30] It reversibly blocks the binding of RANKL to RANK in preosteoclasts and osteoclasts and inhibits the formation, activation, function, activity, and survival of osteoclasts. It does not cross-react with other human proteins of similar structure, and being fully human, its potential to elicit an anti-antibody response is low.[31] Given its specificity, it has few off-target effects. It neither interferes with immune functions, nor predisposes to neoplasia, nor enhances the progression of underlying neoplastic lesions.

A single subcutaneous injection induces a rapid, profound, and sustained dose-dependent inhibition of bone resorption lasting for about 6 months.[32] Unlike bisphosphonates, it is not incorporated in bones.[33] Peak serum concentration is reached 1 to 4 weeks post injection and declines over a 4- to 5-month period to nearly undetectable levels. Its serum half-life is about 26 days. Its inhibitory activity on bone resorption is reversible.[31] Because it is not excreted by the kidneys, it can be administered to patients with impaired renal function. It is contraindicated in patients with hypocalcemia.

Efficacy

- *Postmenopausal women with osteoporosis:* The FREEDOM (Fracture Reduction Evaluation of Denosumab in Osteoporosis every six Months) trial: Over a 3-year period compared with placebo, denosumab reduced the relative risk of hip fractures by 40%, morphometric vertebral fractures by 68%, and nonvertebral fractures by 20%. Compared with placebo, the increases in lumbar spine and total hip BMD were 9.2% and 6.0%, respectively, and the levels of BTMs (CTX) were reduced by 86% by the first month and 72% by 6 months. The study included 7,868 postmenopausal women between the ages of 60 and 90 years with a lumbar spine or total hip T-score of −2.5 or lower, but not lower than −4.0; 23% of the subjects had vertebral compression fractures.[34]

  - Denosumab is effective in patients with impaired renal function: In 73 and 2,817 patients with an estimated creatinine clearance between 15 and 29 mL/minute and 30 to 59 mL/minute, respectively, fracture risk reduction and changes in BMD were similar to those with normal renal function.[35]

  - Denosumab is effective at reducing the incidence of fractures in postmenopausal women at higher risk of fractures because of previous fractures, low BMD (T-scores −3.0 or lower), or advanced age (>70 years).[36]

  - The extension of the FREEDOM study for 2 years included 4,550 patients all on denosumab; the ones who were on placebo during the first 3 years switched to denosumab.[37] In patients who were on denosumab in the first 3 years, continuing denosumab further increased BMD. By the end of the fifth year the BMD had increased by 13.7% in the lumbar vertebrae and 7.0% in the total hip. The reductions in BTMs were maintained in patients who continued with denosumab. Data presented at scientific meetings on 6- and 8-year extensions of the FREEDOM and Phase 2 studies confirm the continued increase in BMD (15.2% and 7.5% by year 6 in the lumbar vertebrae and total hip, respectively) and sustained reduction in BTMs.[38,39]

- *Postmenopausal women with osteopenia:* Over a 24-month period compared with placebo, denosumab significantly increased BMD at the lumbar spine (+6.5% vs. −0.6%), total hip (+3.4% vs. −1.1%), femoral neck (+2.8% vs. −0.9%), trochanter (+5.2% vs. −0.8%), one-third radius (+1.4% vs. −2.1%), and total body (+2.4% vs. −1.4%). The study was conducted on 332 postmenopausal women with osteopenia. The overall incidence of adverse effects was similar in both groups.[40]

- *Cancer-related bone demineralization and osteoporosis:* Denosumab is effective in the management of low bone mass in oncology patients on aromatase inhibitors or androgen deprivation therapy.[39,40]

- *Patients with rheumatoid arthritis:* In patients with rheumatoid arthritis, denosumab protects against bone erosion, reduces bone turnover, and increases BMD.[43]

- *Low bone mineral density in men:* Studies documented the positive effects of denosumab in the management of osteoporosis in men[44] and, in the USA, the FDA approved denosumab to increase bone mass in men with osteoporosis at high risk for fracture.[44]

Adverse Effects

Results of the FREEDOM study show that the subcutaneous injections were well tolerated. Overall rates of adverse events were similar in the denosumab and placebo groups. There were 70 and 90 deaths in the denosumab and placebo groups, respectively. Cellulitis as a serious adverse event, eczema, and flatulence were reported more frequently with denosumab than placebo. There were no differences in the number of patients withdrawing from the study: 17.9% in the placebo group and 16.1% in the denosumab group. No neutralizing antibodies against denosumab were detected. The risk of neoplasia, infections, cardiovascular diseases, and hypocalcemia was not increased. Delayed fracture healing was reported in two patients on denosumab and four on placebo. There were no instances of osteonecrosis of the jaw or atypical femur fractures.[34] A subsequent review of infections occurring during the FREEDOM data pointed toward a heterogenous etiology with no clear relationship between denosumab and infections.[45] In the extension study, adverse events did not increase, but two cases of osteonecrosis of the jaw were reported in patients who had been on placebo during the first 3 years and then switched to denosumab.[37] A further analysis of adverse effects in long-term extension and crossover studies in postmenopausal women with osteoporosis did not show an increased risk of infections (including cellulitis/erysipelas and infective endocarditis), malignancy, or hypocalcemia.[46]

Discontinuation of Denosumab

Discontinuation of denosumab leads to decreases in BMD and increases in BTMs levels. This study was conducted on 256 postmenopausal women with a mean age of 59 years and mean T-score at the lumbar spine −1.6.[47] Histomorphometry studies confirmed that the effects of denosumab on bone turnover are fully reversible.[48]

Denosumab versus Alendronate and Switching from Alendronate to Denosumab

Over a 12-month period compared with alendronate, denosumab induced greater increases in BMD of the total hip (3.5% vs. 2.6%), lumbar vertebrae (5.3% vs. 4.2%), femoral neck (2.4% vs. 1.8%), trochanter (4.5% vs. 3.4%), and distal one-third radius (1.1% vs. 0.6%). Reductions in BTMs were also more pronounced in the denosumab group. The DECIDE Trial (Determining Efficacy: Comparison of Initiating Denosumab versus Alendronate) included 1,189 postmenopausal women with a lumbar or total hip T-score of −2.0 or lower. Overall tolerability was similar in both groups.[49]

Transitioning from alendronate to denosumab leads to greater increases in BMD at the total hip 1.9% versus 1.05% and lumbar vertebrae 3.03% versus 1.85%. Changes in the femoral neck, and distal one-third radius were also more pronounced in the denosumab group. Similarly greater decreases in a BTMs (CTX) were observed in the denosumab group. The Study of Transitioning from Alendronate to Denosumab (STAND) trial included 504 postmenopausal women 55 years of age or older with a T-score of −2.0 or less but −4.0 or higher who had been on alendronate for at least 6 months. They were randomly allocated to either continue with weekly alendronate or switch to denosumab 60 mg subcutaneously. There were no differences in overall adverse effects in both groups.[50] Adherence was better with denosumab than alendronate.[51]

Calcitonin

Calcitonin (synthetic salmon) is available as 200 IU administered by daily intranasal insufflations for the treatment of postmenopausal osteoporosis. Calcitonin, a hormone secreted by the C-cells of the thyroid gland (see Chapter 2), inhibits the activity of osteoclasts, reduces bone resorption, and increases renal calcium excretion. It induces significant decreases in BTMs, reaching nadir at 6 months.[52] Its main adverse effect is nasal irritation. Because the amino acid sequence of salmon calcitonin is different from human calcitonin, its continuous administration leads to the formation of antibodies: 39%, 52%, and 61% of subjects receiving nasal calcitonin develop antibodies after 6, 12, and 18 months, respectively. These antibodies, however, are not neutralizing and do not interfere with the biologic activities of calcitonin.[53]

Efficacy

- *Postmenopausal women with osteoporosis:* The PROOF study (Prevent Recurrence of Osteoporotic Fractures): Over a 5-year period compared with placebo, intranasally-administered salmon calcitonin (200 IU) reduced the risk of new vertebral fractures by 33% and the risk of further vertebral fractures by 36% in those who had one to five prevalent vertebral fractures at enrollment. BTMs decreased and lumbar spine BMD increased. The study included 1,255 postmenopausal women with osteoporosis. Calcitonin was well tolerated.[54]

- *Prevention of osteoporosis in early postmenopausal women:* When administered to postmenopausal women within 3 years of menopause compared with placebo, calcitonin induced significant increases in BMD and decreases in BTMs.[55,56]

- *Post hip fracture and total hip arthroplasty:* The administration of calcitonin to 37 women who had sustained a hip fracture and underwent total hip arthroplasty documented that compared with a control group of 38 women, the rate of refracture and periprosthetic ossification was reduced. Similarly, calcitonin led to greater increases in functional independence.[57]

- *Analgesic effect:* Calcitonin 200 IU administered intranasally to patients who have sustained an acute vertebral compression fracture significantly reduced pain and the need for analgesics when compared with placebo.[58] The daily subcutaneous administration of salmon calcitonin (100 IU) compared with placebo increased the plasma levels of beta-endorphin at the end of 2 weeks. This was associated with pain reduction and improvement in quality of life parameters. The study included 30 patients receiving salmon calcitonin and 26 receiving placebo.[59]

Alternative Methods of Administration

Alternative routes of administration are being studied. The rectal route, although effective, is not tolerated by many patients.[60] The oral route looks promising:[61] When administered to 277 postmenopausal women, it induced dose-dependent decreases in BTMs levels, reaching a nadir 2 to 3 hours post dose administration. It was well tolerated,[62] and large scale multicenter studies were launched. In December 2011, however, Novartis Pharma AG announced it was no longer pursuing the clinical development of oral calcitonin for the management of postmenopausal osteoporosis because it had not met key efficacy end-points.[63]

Selective Estrogen Receptor Modulators: Raloxifene

Raloxifene is available as 60 mg tablets once a day for the treatment and prevention of postmenopausal osteoporosis. Selective estrogen receptor modulators (SERMs) or estrogen agonists/antagonists bind to estrogen receptors alfa (ERα) and beta (ERβ), resulting in conformational changes at the ligand-binding domain that may be similar to or different from estrogen depending on the physiochemical properties of the SERM. The estrogen agonist and antagonist activity of SERM varies according to the expression of coactivators and corepressors of gene activity.

Efficacy

- **Postmenopausal women with osteoporosis:** Over a 3-year period compared with placebo in postmenopausal women with osteoporosis, raloxifene (60 mg and 120 mg once a day) increased BMD at the lumbar spine and femoral neck, decreased BTMs levels, and reduced the risk of vertebral, but not nonvertebral fractures. The 60 mg raloxifene dose reduced the risk of new radiographic vertebral fractures by 30%. The Multiple Outcomes of Raloxifene Evaluation (MORE) trial[64] included 7,705 postmenopausal women with osteoporosis (age 31 to 80 years, mean 67 years) randomized to receive daily oral placebo or raloxifene 60 or 120 mg.

    A 12-month extension of the MORE trial to 4 years showed similar reductions in the risk of vertebral fractures.[65] A further 4-year extension, the Continuing Outcomes Relevant to Evista (CORE) trial,[66] showed that the increases in BMD persisted, but there was no effect on the risk of nonvertebral fractures. The primary objective of the CORE Trial was to evaluate the effect of raloxifene on breast cancer.

Adverse Effects

The risk of venous thromboembolism was increased by about threefold, similar to estrogen replacement therapy. Therefore, raloxifene should not be prescribed to women with an active or past history of venous thromboembolism. There was a small but significant increase in hot flashes and leg cramps with raloxifene. The risk-benefit balance should be carefully considered in women at risk for stroke [67] Raloxifene is also approved for reduction of invasive breast cancer in postmenopausal women at high risk for invasive breast cancer.

Estrogen

In the United States, estrogen is approved for prevention, but not treatment, of postmenopausal osteoporosis. The skeletal benefit of estrogen in postmenopausal women was firmly established by the Women's Health Initiative (WHI) in two large, double-blind, placebo-controlled studies: estrogen plus progestin therapy (EPT)[68] and estrogen therapy (ET) alone for postmenopausal women who had undergone a hysterectomy.[69] Compared with placebo, EPT reduced hip fractures by 36%, clinical vertebral fractures by 36%, and other osteoporotic fractures by 23%. Similarly, ET reduced hip fractures by 39% and clinical vertebral fractures by 38%.[69]

Estrogen—with or without progestin in a variety of doses and formulations—is primarily used in early postmenopausal women for the treatment of menopausal symptoms. When prescribed solely for the prevention of postmenopausal osteoporosis, it should be used for women at significant risk of osteoporosis when nonestrogen medications are not considered appropriate. Treatment decisions should be individualized, using the lowest effective dose of estrogen for the shortest period of time consistent with the goals and potential risks of treatment. Estrogen is most often used in "young" (<age 60) postmenopausal women with low risk for stroke and breast cancer for less than 5 years, but may be appropriate for other patients for a longer duration according to clinical circumstances. Long-term use of estrogen for skeletal health in women without menopausal symptoms may be considered when the risk-benefit balance is favorable. The skeletal benefits of estrogen rapidly dissipate after its discontinuation.

Strontium Ranelate

Strontium ranelate is orally administered and licensed for use in the European Union and other countries, but not the United States and Canada. It is composed of two atoms of stable strontium and an organic moiety, ranelic acid. Evidence for its antifracture efficacy comes from two large trials: Spinal Osteoporosis Therapeutic Intervention (SOTI) study[70] and Treatment of Peripheral Osteoporosis (TROPOS) study.[71] Several smaller studies, including Strontium Ranelate for Treatment of Osteoporosis (STRATOS)[72] and Prevention of Osteoporosis (PREVOS)[73] support its effects on BMD and BTMs.

Although the mechanism of action of strontium is not completely understood, it appears to uncouple the bone remodeling process, increasing bone formation and decreasing bone resorption. The absorption of strontium is competitive with calcium, and once absorbed, strontium has a strong affinity for bone. Because strontium has a higher atomic number ($Z = 38$) than calcium ($Z = 20$), when it replaces calcium in bone, a large increase in BMD occurs despite modest changes in BTMs.[74] BMD is useful in monitoring patients for adherence to therapy with strontium, although the relationship between BMD change and reduction in fracture risk may not be the same as with other medications.

Strontium ranelate is administered orally as a 2 g sachet (packaged granules with 680 mg elemental strontium taken as a suspension in at least 30 mL water) once daily at bedtime, preferably at least 2 hours after eating. The absorption of strontium ranelate is reduced by 60% to 70% if taken with food or medications containing calcium. It is not recommended for patients with severe renal impairment (creatinine clearance <30 mL/minute). No dosage adjustment is necessary for patients with moderate renal impairment. Hypersensitivity reactions, including drug rash with eosinophilia and systemic symptoms (DRESS), sometimes fatal, appeared in postmarketing reports of strontium ranelate, with no clear evidence of causality.

Other forms of strontium (e.g., strontium citrate) are available over the counter. The use of these products for osteoporosis should be discouraged because of lack of data on efficacy and safety.

Therapeutic Agents Under Development

Advances in understanding the pathogenesis of osteoporosis and the regulation of bone remodeling at cellular and molecular levels led to the identification of new potential therapeutic targets. [75]

Cathepsin K Inhibitors

In the process of bone resorption, osteoclasts attach to the bone surface by means of a sealing zone that creates a space between osteoclasts and bone surface isolated from the marrow. This microenvironment is acidified by means of a proton pump that mobilizes bone mineral and exposes the organic collagen matrix. Cysteine proteases, particularly cathepsin K, then degrade the collagen. Cathepsin K is a potential target for the treatment of diseases associated with high bone resorption, including postmenopausal osteoporosis. Compounds that inhibit cathepsin K include balicatib (AAE581, Novartis), relacatib (SB-462795, GlaxoSmithKline), ONO-5334 (Ono Pharma), and odanacatib (MK-0822, MK-822, Merck/Celera). The latter is most advanced in clinical development.

Sclerostin Inhibitiors

Osteocytes appear to have a skeletal mechano-sensing role, with sclerostin being a key signaling protein. Sclerostin is a protein encoded by the SOST gene in osteocytes and other terminally differentiated cells within the bone matrix. It inhibits osteoblast differentiation, activity, and survival by binding to low-density lipoprotein receptor-related proteins 5 and 6 on the cell surface of osteoblasts, thereby antagonizing Wnt/β-catenin signaling. Sclerostin is a potential target for therapeutic intervention in patients with osteoporosis, with inhibition of sclerostin (i.e., downregulating an inhibitor of bone formation) expected to have an osteoanabolic effect. Interestingly, inhibition of sclerostin does not increase bone resorption as is seen with other osteoanabolic agents (e.g., teriparatide and PTH[1–84]). [76] This suggests that inhibition of sclerostin may at least partially uncouple bone formation and resorption, with potential therapeutic effects greater than those of currently approved osteoanabolic agents. AMG 785 (CDP7851, romosozumab; codeveloped by Amgen, Thousand Oaks, CA, USA and UCB, Belgium) is an investigational humanized sclerostin monoclonal antibody undergoing clinical trials. Other antisclerostin compounds are also being evaluated.

Conclusion

A number of medications are now available for the management of osteoporosis. Each has a unique profile. There is no panacea, no single "best medication" for all patients. The comparative efficacy and safety of different medications cannot be established to any degree of certainty: Most large double-blind controlled clinical trials were not done to compare the risk-benefit ratio of different medications but to gain approval from regulatory agencies by comparing active medication to placebo. Because often the diagnostic thresholds, inclusion and exclusion criteria, methodology, and even assessments are different in different studies,[77] it is difficult to use results from clinical trials to compare the efficacy/safety of different medications. Therefore, clinicians must use their judgment and experience to individualize treatment decisions.

References

1. Finkelstein JS, Wyland JJ, Leder BZ, et al. Effects of teriparatide retreatment in osteoporotic men and women. J Clin Endocrinol Metab. 2009;94(7):2495–501.

2. Yu EW, Neer RM, Lee H, et al. Time-dependent changes in skeletal response to teriparatide: escalating vs. constant dose teriparatide (PTH 1–34) in osteoporotic women. Bone. 2011;48(4):713–19.

3. Silva BC, Bilezikian JP. New approaches to the treatment of osteoporosis. Annu Rev Med. 2011;62:307–22.

4. Kaufman JM, Orwoll E, Goemaere S, et al. Teriparatide effects on vertebral fractures and bone mineral density in men with osteoporosis: treatment and discontinuation of therapy. Osteoporos Int. 2005;16(5):510–16.

5. Leder BZ, Neer RM, Wyland JJ, et al. Effects of teriparatide treatment and discontinuation in postmenopausal women and eugonadal men with osteoporosis. J Clin Endocrinol Metab. 2009;94(8):2915–21.

6. Adachi JD, Hanley DA, Lorraine JK, et al. Assessing compliance, acceptance, and tolerability of teriparatide in patients with osteoporosis who fractured while on anti-resorptive treatment or were intolerant to previous anti-resorptive treatment: an 18-month, multicenter, open-label, prospective study. Clin Ther. 2007;29(9):2055–67.

7. Foster SA, Foley KA, Meadows ES, et al. Adherence and persistence with teriparatide among patients with commercial, Medicare, and Medicaid insurance. Osteoporos Int. 2011;22(2):551–57.

8. Daddona PE, Matriano JA, Mandema J, et al. Parathyroid hormone (1–34)-coated microneedle patch system: clinical pharmacokinetics and pharmacodynamics for treatment of osteoporosis. Pharm Res. 2011;28(1):159–65.

9. Neer RM, Arnaud CD, Zanchetta JR, et al. Effect of parathyroid hormone (1–34) on fractures and bone mineral density in postmenopausal women with osteoporosis. N Engl J Med. 2001;344(19):1434–41.

10. Lindsay R, Scheele WH, Neer R, et al. Sustained vertebral fracture risk reduction after withdrawal of teriparatide in postmenopausal women with osteoporosis. Arch Intern Med. 2004;164(18):2024–30.

11. Prince R, Sipos A, Hossain A, et al. Sustained nonvertebral fragility fracture risk reduction after discontinuation of teriparatide treatment. J Bone Miner Res. 2005;20(9):1507–13.

12. Fahrleitner-Pammer A, Langdahl BL, Marin F, et al. Fracture rate and back pain during and after discontinuation of teriparatide: 36-month data from the European Forsteo Observational Study (EFOS). Osteoporos Int. 2011;22(10):2709–19.

13. Maugeri D, Russo E, Luca S, et al. Changes of the quality-of-life under the treatment of severe senile osteoporosis with teriparatide. Arch Gerontol Geriatr. 2009 Jul-;49(1):35–38.

14. Carvalho NN, Voss LA, Almeida MO, et al. Atypical femoral fractures during prolonged use of bisphosphonates: short-term responses to strontium ranelate and teriparatide. J Clin Endocrinol Metab. 2011;96(9):2675–80.

15. Oteo-Álvaro Á, Matas JA, Alonso-Farto JC. Teriparatide (rh [1–34] PTH) improved osteointegration of a hemiarthroplasty with signs of aseptic loosening. Orthopedics. 2011;34(9):e574–77.

16. Bashutski JD, Eber RM, Kinney JS, et al. Teriparatide and osseous regeneration in the oral cavity. N Engl J Med. 2010;363(25):2396–405.

17. Hellmeyer L, Boekhoff J, Hadji P. Treatment with teriparatide in a patient with pregnancy-associated osteoporosis. Gynecol Endocrinol. 2010;26(10):725–28.

18. Nogueira EL, Costa AC, Santana A, et al. Teriparatide efficacy in the treatment of severe hypocalcemia after kidney transplantation in parathyroidectomized patients: a series of five case reports. Transplantation. 2011;92(3):316–20.

19. Horowitz BS, Horowitz ME, Fonseca S, et al. An 18-month open-label trial of teriparatide in patients with previous parathyroidectomy at continued risk for osteoporotic fractures: an exploratory study. Endocr Pract. 2011;17(3):377–83.

20. Bilezikian JP, Rubin MR. Combination/sequential therapies for anabolic and anti-resorptive skeletal agents for osteoporosis. Curr Osteoporos Rep. 2006;4(1):5–13.

21. Kurland ES, Heller SL, Diamond B, et al. The importance of bisphosphonate therapy in maintaining bone mass in men after therapy with teriparatide [human parathyroid hormone(1–34)]. Osteoporos Int. 2004;15(12):992–97.

22. Adami S, San Martin J, Muñoz-Torres M, et al. Effect of raloxifene after recombinant teriparatide [hPTH(1–34)] treatment in postmenopausal women with osteoporosis. Osteoporos Int. 2008;19(1):87–94.

23. Black DM, Greenspan SL, Ensrud KE, et al. The effects of parathyroid hormone and alendronate alone or in combination in postmenopausal osteoporosis. N Engl J Med. 2003;349(13):1207–15.

24. Cusano NE, Bilezikian JP. Combination anti-resorptive and osteo-anabolic therapy for osteoporosis: we are not there yet. Curr Med Res Opin. 2011;27(9):1705–07.

25. Cosman F, Eriksen EF, Recknor C, et al. Effects of intravenous zoledronic acid plus subcutaneous teriparatide [rhPTH(1–34)] in postmenopausal osteoporosis. J Bone Miner Res. 2011;26(3):503–11.

26. Deal C, Omizo M, Schwartz EN, et al. Combination teriparatide and raloxifene therapy for postmenopausal osteoporosis: results from a 6-month double-blind placebo-controlled trial. J Bone Miner Res. 2005;20(11):1905–11.

27. Cosman F, Wermers RA, Recknor C, et al. Effects of teriparatide in postmenopausal women with osteoporosis on prior alendronate or raloxifene: differences

between stopping and continuing the anti-resorptive agent. J Clin Endocrinol Metab. 2009;94(10):3772–80.

28. FORTEO® [package insert] Indianapolis, IN: Eli Lilly and Company; 2010.

29. Kendler DL, Bessette L, Hill CD, et al. Preference and satisfaction with a 6-month subcutaneous injection versus a weekly tablet for treatment of low bone mass. Osteoporos Int. 2010;21(5):837–46.

30. Bekker PJ, Holloway DL, Rasmussen AS, et al. A single-dose placebo-controlled study of AMG 162, a fully human monoclonal antibody to RANKL, in postmeno-pausal women. J Bone Miner Res. 2004;19(7):1059–66.

31. Singer A, Gruaer A. Denosumab for the management of postmenopausal osteo-porosis. Postgrad Med 2010;122:176–87.

32. Hamdy NA. Targeting the RANK/RANKL/OPG signaling pathway: a novel approach in the management of osteoporosis. Curr Opin Investig Drugs. 2007;8(4):299–303.

33. Baron R, Ferrari S, Russell RG. Denosumab and bisphosphonates: different mechanisms of action and effects. Bone. 2011;48(4):677–92.

34. Cummings SR, San Martin J, McClung MR, et al. Denosumab for prevention of fractures in postmenopausal women with osteoporosis. N Engl J Med. 2009;361(8):756–65.

35. Jamal SA, Ljunggren O, Stehman-Breen C, et al. Effects of denosumab on frac-ture and bone mineral density by level of kidney function. J Bone Miner Res. 2011;26(8):1829–35.

36. Boonen S, Adachi JD, Man Z, et al. Treatment with denosumab reduces the incidence of new vertebral and hip fractures in postmenopausal women at high risk. J Clin Endocrinol Metab. 2011;96(6):1727–36.

37. Papapoulos S, Chapurlat R, Libanati C, et al. Five years of denosumab exposure in women with postmenopausal osteoporosis: Results from the first two years of the FREEDOM extension. J Bone Miner Res 2012;27(3):694–701.

38. Brown JP, Bone HG, Chapurlat R, et al. Six years of denosumab treatment in postmenopausal women with osteoporosis: results from the first three years of the FREEDOM extension. Presented at ACR; Chicago; November, 2011.

39. McClung MR, Lewiecki EM, Bolognese MA, et al. Effects of denosumab on bone mineral density and biochemical markers of bone turnover: 8-year results of a phase 2 clinical trial. Presented at ASBMR; San Diego, September 2011.

40. Bone HG, Bolognese MA, Yuen CK, et al. Effects of denosumab on bone mineral density and bone turnover in postmenopausal women. J Clin Endocrinol Metab. 2008;93(6):2149–57.

41. Ellis GK, Bone HG, Chlebowski R, et al. Randomized trial of denosumab in patients receiving adjuvant aromatase inhibitors for nonmetastatic breast can-cer. J Clin Oncol. 2008;26(30):4875–82.

42. Smith MR, Egerdie B, Hernández Toriz N, et al. Denosumab in men receiv-ing androgen-deprivation therapy for prostate cancer. N Engl J Med. 2009;361(8):745–55.

43. Deodhar A, Dore RK, Mandel D, et al. Denosumab-mediated increase in hand bone mineral density associated with decreased progression of bone erosion in rheumatoid arthritis patients. Arthritis Care Res (Hoboken). 2010;62(4):569–74.

44. Orwoll E, Teglbjaerg CS, Langdahl BL, et al. A randomized, placebo-controlled study of the effects of denosumab for the treatment of men with low bone min-eral density. J Clin Endocrin Metab 2012;97(9):3161–3169

45. Watts NB, Roux C, Modlin JF, et al. Infections in postmenopausal women with osteoporosis treated with denosumab or placebo: coincidence or causal association? Osteoporos Int 2012;23:327–37.

46. Bone HG, Chapurlat R, Libanati C, et al. Safety observations from denosumab long-term extension and cross-over studies in postmenopausal women with osteoporosis. Presented at ASBMR, San Diego, September 2011.

47. Bone HG, Bolognese MA, Yuen CK, et al. Effects of denosumab treatment and discontinuation on bone mineral density and bone turnover markers in postmenopausal women with low bone mass. J Clin Endocrinol Metab. 2011;96(4):972–80.

48. Brown JP, Dempster DW, Ding B, et al. Bone remodeling in postmenopausal women who discontinued denosumab treatment: off-treatment biopsy study. J Bone Miner Res. 2011;26(11):2737–44.

49. Brown JP, Prince RL, Deal C, et al. Comparison of the effect of denosumab and alendronate on BMD and biochemical markers of bone turnover in postmenopausal women with low bone mass: a randomized, blinded, phase 3 trial. J Bone Miner Res. 2009;24(1):153–61.

50. Kendler DL, Roux C, Benhamou CL, et al. Effects of denosumab on bone mineral density and bone turnover in postmenopausal women transitioning from alendronate therapy. J Bone Miner Res. 2010;25(1):72–81.

51. Freemantle N, Satram-Hoang S, Tang ET, et al. Final results of the DAPS (Denosumab Adherence Preference Satisfaction) study: a 24-month, randomized, crossover comparison with alendronate in postmenopausal women. Osteoporos Int. 2012;23(1):317–26.

52. Srivastava AK, Libanati C, Hohmann O, et al. Acute effects of calcitonin nasal spray on serum C-telopeptide of type 1 collagen (CTx) levels in elderly osteopenic women with increased bone turnover. Calcif Tissue Int. 2004;75(6):477–81.

53. Reginster JY, Gaspar S, Deroisy R, et al. Prevention of osteoporosis with nasal salmon calcitonin: effect of anti-salmon calcitonin antibody formation. Osteoporos Int. 1993;3(5):261–64.

54. Chesnut CH 3rd, Silverman S, Andriano K, et al. A randomized trial of nasal spray salmon calcitonin in postmenopausal women with established osteoporosis: the prevent recurrence of osteoporotic fractures study. PROOF Study Group. Am J Med. 2000;109(4):267–76.

55. Overgaard K. Effect of intranasal salmon calcitonin therapy on bone mass and bone turnover in early postmenopausal women: a dose-response study. Calcif Tissue Int. 1994;55(2):82–86.

56. Arnala I, Saastamoinen J, Alhava EM. Salmon calcitonin in the prevention of bone loss at perimenopause. Bone. 1996;18(6):629–32.

57. Peichl P, Marteau R, Griesmacher A, et al. Salmon calcitonin nasal spray treatment for postmenopausal women after hip fracture with total hip arthroplasty. J Bone Miner Metab. 2005;23(3):243–52.

58. Lyritis GP, Paspati I, Karachalios T, et al. Pain relief from nasal salmon calcitonin in osteoporotic vertebral crush fractures. A double blind, placebo-controlled clinical study. Acta Orthop Scand Suppl. 1997;275:112–14.

59. Ofluoglu D, Akyuz G, Unay O, et al. The effect of calcitonin on beta-endorphin levels in postmenopausal osteoporotic patients with back pain. Clin Rheumatol. 2007;26(1):44–49.

60. Lyritis GP, Ioannidis GV, Karachalios T, et al. Analgesic effect of salmon calcitonin suppositories in patients with acute pain due to recent osteoporotic vertebral crush fractures: a prospective double-blind, randomized, placebo-controlled clinical study. Clin J Pain. 1999;15(4):284–89.

61. Karsdal MA, Henriksen K, Bay-Jensen AC, et al. Lessons learned from the development of oral calcitonin: the first tablet formulation of a protein in phase III clinical trials. J Clin Pharmacol 2011;51:460–71.

62. Tankó LB, Bagger YZ, Alexandersen P, et al. Safety and efficacy of a novel salmon calcitonin (sCT) technology-based oral formulation in healthy postmenopausal women: acute and 3-month effects on biomarkers of bone turnover. J Bone Miner Res. 2004;19(9):1531–38.

63. Hamdy RC, Daley D. Oral Calcitonin. Int J Women's Health. 2012;4;471–79.

64. Ettinger B, Black DM, Mitlak BH, et al. Reduction of vertebral fracture risk in postmenopausal women with osteoporosis treated with raloxifene: results from a 3-year randomized clinical trial. Multiple Outcomes of Raloxifene Evaluation (MORE) Investigators. JAMA. 1999;282(7):637–45.

65. Delmas PD, Ensrud KE, Adachi JD, et al. Efficacy of raloxifene on vertebral fracture risk reduction in postmenopausal women with osteoporosis: four-year results from a randomized clinical trial. J Clin Endocrinol Metab. 2002;87(8):3609–17.

66. Martino S, Cauley JA, Barrett-Connor E, et al. Continuing outcomes relevant to Evista: breast cancer incidence in postmenopausal osteoporotic women in a randomized trial of raloxifene. J Natl Cancer Inst. 2004;96(23):1751–61.

67. Barrett-Connor E, Mosca L, Collins P, et al. Effects of raloxifene on cardiovascular events and breast cancer in postmenopausal women. N Engl J Med. 2006;355(2):125–37.

68. Rossouw JE, Anderson GL, Prentice RL, et al. Risks and benefits of estrogen plus progestin in healthy postmenopausal women: principal results From the Women's Health Initiative randomized controlled trial. JAMA. 2002;288(3):321–33.

69 Anderson GL, Limacher M, Assaf AR, et al. Effects of conjugated equine estrogen in postmenopausal women with hysterectomy: the Women's Health Initiative randomized controlled trial. JAMA. 2004;291(14):1701–12.

70. Meunier PJ, Roux C, Seeman E, et al. The effects of strontium ranelate on the risk of vertebral fracture in women with postmenopausal osteoporosis. N Engl J Med. 2004;350(5):459–68.

71. Reginster JY, Seeman E, De Vernejoul MC, et al. Strontium ranelate reduces the risk of nonvertebral fractures in postmenopausal women with osteoporosis: Treatment of Peripheral Osteoporosis (TROPOS) study. J Clin Endocrinol Metab. 2005;90(5):2816–22.

72. Meunier PJ, Slosman DO, Delmas PD, et al. Strontium ranelate: dose-dependent effects in established postmenopausal vertebral osteoporosis--a 2-year randomized placebo controlled trial. J Clin Endocrinol Metab. 2002;87(5):2060–66.

73. Reginster JY, Deroisy R, Dougados M, et al. Prevention of early postmenopausal bone loss by strontium ranelate: the randomized, two-year, double-masked, dose-ranging, placebo-controlled PREVOS trial. Osteoporos Int. 2002;13(12):925–31.

74. Blake GM, Lewiecki EM, Kendler DL, et al. A review of strontium ranelate and its effect on DXA scans. J Clin Densitom. 2007;10(2):113–19.

75. Lewiecki EM. New targets for intervention in the treatment of postmenopausal osteoporosis. Nat Rev Rheumatol. 2011;7:631–38.

76. Ominsky MS, Vlasseros F, Jolette J, et al. Two doses of sclerostin antibody in cynomolgus monkeys increases bone formation, bone mineral density, and bone strength. J Bone Miner Res. 2010;25(5):948–59.

77. Hamdy RC, Price DM, Mottl MM. Diagnostic thresholds in osteoporosis: how are they used in clinical trials? Curr Osteoporos Rep 2011;9(3):160–66.

Chapter 9

Monitoring Patients on Treatment

The desired clinical outcome of treating patients with osteoporosis is no fracture. No drug, however, can completely eliminate the risk of fractures, because fractures are stochastic events depending on whether a patient falls, is subjected to trauma, the force applied to bone, and bone strength. Because no test directly measures bone strength in vivo, clinicians rely on surrogate measurements to evaluate response to therapy.

The results obtained in clinical trials are not always seen in clinical practice, partly because patients often differ from clinical trial subjects in terms of age, other disease states, concomitant medications, and adherence to therapy. Many patients meeting standard indications for treatment of osteoporosis would not qualify for participation in studies required to obtain regulatory approval.[1] Furthermore, because the number of patients included in clinical trials is relatively small, uncommon or rare adverse effects may not be recognized in trials, yet are seen in clinical practice.

Any medication is only effective if taken as prescribed. Adherence is often problematic with medications on a long-term basis for essentially asymptomatic conditions. Therefore, the patient, should be monitored to ensure adherence, efficacy, and be vigilant about adverse drug effects. The main tools available to monitor patients' response are listed below.

Bone Turnover Markers

Monitoring response to therapy is arguably the best validated clinical application of bone turnover markers (BTMs), and clinicians can evaluate drug effect sooner than with dual-energy x-ray absorptiometry (DXA).[2,3] Several markers of bone resorption are available, the most commonly used ones include fasting serum C-telopeptide (CTX), serum N-telopeptide (NTX), and urinary NTX (see Chapter 2). A decrease in a BTM is a measure of therapeutic efficacy of antiresorptive agents, is predictive of subsequent increases in bone mineral density (BMD)[4] and reduction in fracture risk,[5,6] and reinforces patient compliance.[7] The objective is to reduce BTM levels to the premenopausal reference range. Absence of anticipated BTM response suggests a need for further evaluation and reassessment of treatment.[3]

DXA Scans

DXA is commonly used to monitor treatment effect because of its widespread accessibility, low cost, excellent precision, low radiation, and common usage in clinical trials (see Chapter 3). Quantitative ultrasound is not recommended for monitoring therapy because the change in measured parameters is too slow to be clinically useful.[8] Quantitative computed tomography can be used to monitor BMD changes over time, but is not often used in clinical practice because of its high cost and greater exposure to ionizing radiation compared with DXA.

Changes in BMD versus Changes in T-scores

The absolute BMD (in g/cm^2), not T-scores, should be used when monitoring patients' response to therapy (see Chapter 3).

BMD Changes and Fracture Risk

The magnitude of BMD changes induced by different medications varies according to medication used and the individual patient (see Chapters 7 and 8). The greatest increase is typically seen in the first year(s) of therapy, and is followed by a slower increase. Larger increases in BMD are associated with greater reductions in the risk of nonvertebral fractures.[9] Other factors, however, modulate the fracture risk.[10] A Poisson regression model predicted that an increase in lumbar spine BMD of 8% would reduce vertebral fracture risk by 54%, with only 41% of risk reduction explained by BMD increases.[11]

Same Densitometer

Serial BMD tests should be with the same bone densitometer. Quantitative comparison of BMD measured with different bone densitometers cannot be made unless cross-calibration has been done. Details about cross-calibration techniques can be found on the ISCD website and the websites of densitometer manufacturers (see Chapter 3).

Precision and Least Significant Change

The clinical utility of BMD testing to monitor therapy requires strict adherence to quality standards, performance of precision assessment, calculation of least significant change (LSC), and training of DXA technologists and interpreters.[12] Frequent phantom scanning is used to assess the accuracy and stability of BMD measurements. Patient positioning should be correct and consistent in order to obtain accurate and comparable measurements. Precision assessment is necessary to distinguish between measurement errors and BMD changes that are likely to be meaningful. Precision assessment is typically conducted by measuring BMD in 15 patients three times or 30 patients twice each, with repositioning of the patient after each scan. The values obtained are used to calculate the LSC, the smallest change in BMD (expressed as g/cm^2) that is statistically significant, usually with a 95% level of confidence.

The LSC supplied by the DXA manufacturer cannot be used for individual patients because it may be different and is often better than LSC in clinical settings.

Best Skeletal Site to Scan

The best skeletal site for monitoring response to therapy is one that responds quickly to therapy and has low LSC. For most patients, the lumbar spine is the preferred site to monitor. When the lumbar spine is not evaluable (e.g., owing to degenerative arthritis or other artifacts), the total hip is often used.

An acceptable response to therapy is stability or increase in BMD; both have been associated with reductions in fracture risk in clinical trials. About 10%

of clinical practice patients treated with a bisphosphonate have a statistically significant decrease in BMD, often caused by previously unrecognized contributing factors.[13]

Individualizing the Follow-up of Patients Prescribed Medication to Reduce Fracture Risk

The follow-up of patients prescribed medications for osteoporosis depends on the severity of the condition, the prescribed medication, the patient's individual circumstances, and the practice type. The following protocol is suggested.

Initial Visit(s): Motivate and Educate Patients

Diagnostic classification (e.g., osteoporosis, osteopenia, normal) is established, fracture risk assessed, and secondary causes of bone demineralization excluded at the time of the initial visit(s). If antiresorptive therapy is contemplated, the patient's gums are checked for exposed bone. It may be prudent to postpone antiresorptive therapy until any planned invasive dental procedure is completed and healed.

Patients need to appreciate the seriousness of their condition, the consequences not being treated, the expected benefits and potential risks of pharmacological therapy. The importance of healthy lifestyle and good nutrition should be discussed. Patient education and motivation are essential. Regrettably, the media, which tend to publicize the rare and sensational, may have a negative impact on patient adherence with the prescribed medication. The FRAX® estimation of fracture risk helps patients appreciate the magnitude of risk and the risk-benefit ratio of the prescribed medication. The management strategy should include calcium and vitamin D intake, and lifestyle changes such as

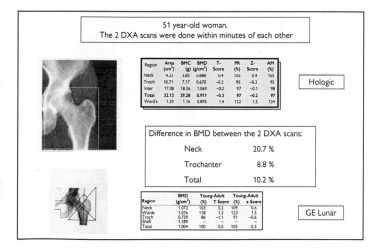

Figure 9.1 Follow-Up Should Be Done with the Same Densitometer. These Two Scans were Done on the Same Patient a Few Minutes Apart. Note the Different BMD Values as well as T-Scores and z-Scores.

reducing sodium (salt, soda drinks) and caffeine intake, discontinuing cigarette smoking, and if possible enrolling in an exercise program.

Initial Follow-up Visit

- **Parenterally administered medications: intravenous bisphospho-nates or subcutaneous denosumab—4 to 6 weeks:** This visit addresses any experienced adverse effect(s) and ensures that recommended lifestyle changes have been made. The patient is reminded of the next administration and necessary blood tests. The informed patient who knows she has an appointment scheduled is less likely to contact the office unnecessarily.

- **Teriparatide—6 to 8 weeks:** In addition to addressing adverse effects and lifestyle changes, an increase in BTM levels (bone-specific alkaline phosphatase, or P1NP) is predictive of subsequent increases in BMD, helps convince the patient that the daily subcutaneous injections are working and provide motivation to adhere to the medication.[14]

- **Orally administered bisphosphonates—8 to 12 weeks:** This visit helps compliance and addresses adverse effects that may have developed. It also emphasizes the seriousness of the condition, cements the doctor–patient relationship, and is an opportunity to further address lifestyle changes. Assaying a BTM (CTX or NTX) during this visit may convince the patient and reassure the clinician that the medication has reduced bone turnover or may signal noncompliance or secondary osteoporosis.

Subsequent Follow-up Visits During Year 1

Regular follow-up visits help adherence with the medication and recommended lifestyle changes. An alternative to these visits could be phone calls or e-mails from the clinician's office. The patient's compliance is likely to improve if the clinician cares sufficiently to regularly enquire about adherence with the medication and lifestyle changes. The frequency of subsequent follow-up visits is determined individually.

1-Year Follow-up Visit

A 1-year follow-up visit gives an opportunity to systematically review and fine tune the management strategy, renew the prescription, and ensure adherence with the medication and lifestyle changes. The following tests may be considered: serum vitamin D and comprehensive metabolic profile; BTM; and DXA scan. The main goal of a 1-year DXA scan is to detect decreases in BMD that will alert clinicians to secondary causes of osteoporosis or nonadherence. Sharing results with patients may help adherence and lifestyle changes.

Follow-up Visits During Year 2

By the second year of treatment, patients should have adopted a certain routine to ensure adherence with the medication and lifestyle changes. Therefore, the follow-up visits depend on the circumstances of individual patients. Phone calls and e-mails may suffice. Patients on denosumab should have their serum calcium level assayed before each 6-month subcutaneous injection to ensure there is no hypocalcemia. Similarly, patients on zoledronic acid or ibandronate should have their serum calcium assayed and creatinine clearance estimated. Zoledronic acid and ibandronate should not be administered if the glomerular filtration rate is less than 35 and 30 mL/minute, respectively.

2-Year Visit

This visit gives an opportunity to reassess bone mass and monitor the patients' progress. The following may be considered: serum vitamin D; comprehensive metabolic profile; BTM; and DXA scan. If a decrease in BMD is observed, the patient's condition needs to be re-evaluated to ensure adherence with the medication and lifestyle changes and rule out secondary causes of osteoporosis. If the patient has been on teriparatide for a lifetime total of 24 months, it should be discontinued and an antiresorptive prescribed to avoid the loss of BMD accrued during teriparatide therapy.

2- to 4-Year Visits

The following may be considered during these visits: annual assay of the serum vitamin D level and comprehensive metabolic profile; BTM; and a DXA scan at 2-year intervals to monitor the BMD. Any significant decrease in BMD should prompt the clinician to enquire about adherence with the medication, lifestyle changes, and to search for secondary causes of osteoporosis.

5-Year Visit

The expected benefits of any medication must be weighed against potential risks. As a general rule, the longer a medication is administered, the higher the risks of adverse effects. Administering antiresorptives for 5 years is associated with significant reductions in fracture risk and relatively few adverse effects. Discontinuing bisphosphonates after 5 years of therapy is associated with an increased fracture risk if the T-score is –2.5 or lower (see Chapter 7). The 5-year mark is an appropriate, although arbitrary, time to re-evaluate the patient and determine whether the medication should be continued. Apart from enquiring about adherence with the prescribed medication, lifestyle changes, and potential adverse effects, the 5-year evaluation of patients on antiresorptives includes the patients':

- *Symptomatology:* Pain in the groin or thighs worsened by standing on the affected leg and associated bone tenderness may suggest a stress or insufficiency fracture that can potentially lead to a full fracture: the atypical femoral shaft fracture (see Chapter 16). Pain in the oral cavity may occur with osteonecrosis of the jaw (see Chapter 17).

- *Changes in BMD:* A continuous increase or stability in BMD suggests a beneficial response to the prescribed medication; therefore, unless there are adverse effects, the medication should be continued and the patient's BMD monitored at 1 to 2-year intervals, especially if the T-score is –2.5 or lower.

- A significant decrease (i.e., BMD change equaling or exceeding the calculated LSC) suggests the patient has an underlying secondary cause for osteoporosis, inadequate calcium and/or vitamin D intake, is not taking the medication regularly or correctly, or has stopped responding to it. If the patient is complying with the intake of the medication, low bone turnover should be considered and a marker of bone resorption assayed. A very low level should prompt the discontinuation of the antiresorptive agent and a re-evaluation 1 year later. Teriparatide may be considered, provided the patient has not already been on this medication.

- **Serum vitamin D level:** A low serum vitamin D level should prompt appropriate replacement.
- **Serum BTM:** Measurement of a BTM is probably not helpful if a favorable BMD response has been demonstrated.

Bisphosphonate Drug Holiday

The concept of a bisphosphonate drug holiday has gained acceptance over the past few years. It is based on limited scientific data for efficacy with long-term treatment (beyond 3 to 5 years) and concern regarding potential adverse outcomes of long-term treatment, especially osteonecrosis of the jaw and atypical femoral fractures[15] (see Chapters 7, 16, and 17). The rationale for a bisphosphonate drug holiday is that the antiresorptive effect and anti-fracture efficacy may continue for a period of time (perhaps 1 or more years) after stopping drug administration due to bisphosphonate retained in the skeleton, while the risk of adverse effects (e.g., osteonecrosis of the jaw and atypical femur fractures) may be reduced. Drug holidays are not appropriate for non-bisphosphonate agents because the beneficial effects of therapy rapidly diminish with discontinuation. In patients on long-term bisphosphonate therapy at high risk of fracture, such as those with a T-score of -2.5 or lower, the benefits of continuing therapy appear to outweigh the risks (see Chapter 7).

Consideration of initiating a bisphosphonate drug holiday should be based on the clinical circumstances and preferences of the patient in the context of the balance of benefit and risk. Patients who are candidates for a drug holiday are those who have been treated with a bisphosphonate for at least 3 to 5 years and are no longer at high risk for fracture. Patients on a drug holiday must be monitored periodically with BMD testing and/or BTMs, with reassessment of fracture risk. When fracture risk is again high, treatment with a bisphosphonate or other agent should be offered.

References

1. Dowd R, Recker RR, Heaney RP. Study subjects and ordinary patients. Osteoporos Int. 2000;11(6):533–36.

2. Lewiecki EM, Baim S, Bilezikian JP, et al. 2008 Santa Fe Bone Symposium: update on osteoporosis. J Clin Densitom. 2009;12(2):135–57.

3. Lewiecki EM, Watts NB. Assessing response to osteoporosis therapy. Osteoporos Int. 2008;19(10):1363–68.

4. Greenspan SL, Parker RA, Ferguson L, et al. Early changes in biochemical markers of bone turnover predict the long-term response to alendronate therapy in representative elderly women: a randomized clinical trial. J Bone Miner Res. 1998;13(9):1431–38.

5. Bauer DC, Black DM, Garnero P, et al. Change in bone turnover and hip, non-spine, and vertebral fracture in alendronate-treated women: the fracture intervention trial. J Bone Miner Res. 2004;19(8):1250–58.

6. Sarkar S, Reginster JY, Crans GG, et al. Relationship between changes in biochemical markers of bone turnover and BMD to predict vertebral fracture risk. J Bone Miner Res. 2004;19(3):394–401.

7. Bergmann P, Body JJ, Boonen S, et al. Evidence-based guidelines for the use of biochemical markers of bone turnover in the selection and monitoring of bis-phosphonate treatment in osteoporosis: a consensus document of the Belgian Bone Club. Int J Clin Pract. 2009;63(1):19–26.

8. Lewiecki EM, Richmond B, Miller PD. Uses and misuses of quantitative ultra-sonography in managing osteoporosis. Cleve Clin J Med. 2006;73(8):742–6, 749–52.

9. Hochberg MC, Greenspan S, Wasnich RD, et al. Changes in bone density and turnover explain the reductions in incidence of nonvertebral fractures that occur during treatment with anti-resorptive agents. J Clin Endocrinol Metab. 2002;87(4):1586–92.

10. Cummings SR, Karpf DB, Harris F, et al. Improvement in spine bone density and reduction in risk of vertebral fractures during treatment with anti-resorptive drugs. Am J Med. 2002;112(4):281–89.

11. Wasnich RD, Miller PD. Antifracture efficacy of anti-resorptive agents are related to changes in bone density. J Clin Endocrinol Metab. 2000;85(1):231–36.

12. Lewiecki EM, Binkley N, Petak SM. DXA quality matters. J Clin Densitom. 2006;9(4):388–92.

13. Lewiecki EM, Rudolph LA. How common is loss of bone mineral density in elderly clinical practice patients receiving oral bisphosphonate therapy for osteoporosis? J Bone Miner Res 2002;17(Suppl 2):S367.

14. Chen P, Satterwhite JH, Licata AA, et al. Early changes in biochemical markers of bone formation predict BMD response to teriparatide in postmenopausal women with osteoporosis. J Bone Miner Res. 2005;20(6):962–70.

15. Bonnick SL. Going on a drug holiday? J Clin Densitom. 2011;14(4):377–83.

Chapter 10

Vertebral Augmentation Procedures

Vertebral fractures are the most common osteoporotic fractures, affecting about 1.4 million individuals each year worldwide.[1] The clinical consequences of vertebral fractures include reduced pulmonary function, chronic back pain, decreased height, kyphosis, loss of self-esteem, abdominal discomfort, disability, and loss of independence, with an increase in mortality of about 20% 5 years after a clinical vertebral fracture.[2,3] The presence of a vertebral fracture increases the risk of future vertebral fractures and other fragility fractures: 19% of patients with an acute vertebral fracture sustain another vertebral fracture within 12 months.[4] The National Osteoporosis Foundation recommends that postmenopausal women and men age 50 and older with a prior vertebral fracture be treated with medication to reduce fracture risk regardless of bone mineral density (BMD).[5]

Conservative medical management of acute painful vertebral fractures consists of rest, analgesics, and sometimes external back bracing, with fracture healing and resolution of pain occurring over the next 6 to 8 weeks in most patients. Unlike treatment of other fractures, traditionally there has been no attempt to correct the fracture deformity, leaving patients with loss of vertebral height that could ultimately result in kyphosis and impaired pulmonary function. For patients with severe pain, hospitalization and narcotic analgesics may be required. Some patients need prolonged bed rest owing to persistence of pain. Potential adverse effects of medical treatment are sedation, impaired cognition, and increased risk of falling. Prolonged bed rest may result in bone loss and muscle weakness.

Because of the limitations of conservative medical treatment and persistence of back pain in some patients, other approaches to management have emerged. Rarely, posterior or lateral displacement of fractured bone fragments compress the spinal cord or nerve roots, requiring urgent surgical intervention with metal implants. Minimally invasive vertebral augmentation procedures involving the percutaneous injection of filler material into the fractured vertebral body have generated considerable interest since the mid-1980s when this procedure was first reported. Subsequently, numerous uncontrolled retrospective case series described rapid pain relief in patients with acute and chronic vertebral fractures. The anecdotal experience of many physicians has been equally impressive. Questions, however, remained concerning the long-term benefits and risks of vertebral augmentation, highlighting the need for high-quality data in long-term randomized controlled trials. In 2011, the Fracture Working Group of the International Osteoporosis Foundation (IOF) published an exhaustive review of prospective controlled studies comparing efficacy and safety of vertebroplasty and kyphoplasty with conservative medical therapy.[2]

Vertebroplasty

Vertebroplasty involves the percutaneous insertion of a needle into a vertebral body and injection of bone cement (usually polymethylmethacrylate, but other filler materials are sometimes used) under high pressure with fluoroscopic guidance. The IOF review identified four prospective nonrandomized studies, two prospective randomized studies, and two prospective randomized single-blind studies. Buchbinder et al. randomized 78 patients (out of 468 screened) with one or two painful vertebral fractures to have vertebroplasty or a simulated sham procedure.[6] There was reduction in pain scores in both groups, with no significant difference between groups at 3 months. No benefit of vertebroplasty over the sham procedure was seen at other time points (1 week, 1 month, and 6 months). Kallmes et al. randomized 131 patients (out of 1831 screened) with one to three painful vertebral fractures to have vertebroplasty or a simulated procedure.[7] The primary outcome measures were disability questionnaire scores and patients' rating of pain intensity at 1 month. It was reported that there was an immediate and sustained improvement with both procedures, but no significant difference between groups. The unexpected findings of these two studies, which have many limitations, received intense scrutiny and generated great controversy. The IOF review concluded that, despite these findings, vertebroplasty provides quicker pain relief and mobility recovery than conservative medical therapy, and that further study with standardized health outcome measures is needed to fully understand the long-term benefits and risks of vertebroplasty (Fig. 10.1).

Kyphoplasty

Kyphoplasty is similar to vertebroplasty, except that injection of the filler material is preceded by the creation of a cavity inside the vertebral body with a balloon tamp (e.g., KyphX Xpander®, KyphX®Exact™; Medtronic, Sunnyvale, CA). The balloon tamp is then withdrawn and bone cement injected into the cavity. This is done under lower pressure and with cement that has a thicker consistency than with vertebroplasty, allowing for a more controlled injection with less risk of leakage beyond the vertebral body than vertebroplasty. The balloon tamp compresses the surrounding trabecular bone and may elevate the fractured vertebral endplates, restoring lost vertebral height in some patients. The IOF review identified one prospective randomized controlled study of kyphoplasty. The Fracture Reduction Evaluation (FREE) trial randomized 300 patients (out of 1,279 screened) with vertebral fractures occurring in the previous 5 to 6 weeks to receive kyphoplasty or nonsurgical care.[8] The primary outcome was the change from baseline to 1 month in the short form physical component summary score, a validated global quality-of-life measure weighted on physical abilities. The group treated with kyphoplasty was found to have significantly higher scores at 1 month compared with the control group. The short-term benefit persisted at 6 months but lost statistical significance at 12 and 24 months,[9] primarily because the nonsurgical group improved with time, probably because of fracture healing. Back pain scores were reduced in both groups compared with

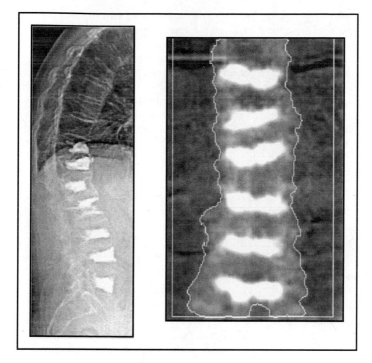

Figure 10.1 Multiple kyphoplasties.

baseline, but reduced significantly more in the kyphoplasty group compared with the control group at all time points from 1 week to 24 months. The IOF review concluded that kyphoplasty provides quicker pain relief and mobility recovery than conservative medical therapy, and that further study is needed.

In some patients undergoing kyphoplasty, restoration of vertebral height achieved by inflation of the balloon tamp is partially lost when the balloon is deflated. One approach to maximizing vertebral height restoration is vertebral body stenting. With this procedure, a metal mesh stent in mounted on a balloon tamp catheter that is expanded inside the vertebral body. The expanded stent remains in place after deflation and removal of the balloon, providing a scaffold to maintain the full volume of the cavity for subsequent injection of the filler material. Results of this procedure are promising,[10,11] but more studies are needed.

Clinical Issues with Vertebral Augmentation

Indications

Patients with painful osteoporotic vertebral fractures who have not responded to conventional medical therapy after 6 to 8 weeks and patients who are immobile owing to severe acute vertebral fracture pain are potential candidates for vertebral augmentation. The finding of spinous process tenderness to palpation at the same level that the fracture deformity is seen on imaging provides supporting evidence that the vertebral body is the source of the back pain.

The Standards of Practice Committee of the Society of Interventional Radiology developed consensus guidelines, using a modified Delphi technique[12] with the following indications for vertebroplasty:[13] painful primary and secondary osteoporotic vertebral compression fracture(s) refractory to medical therapy; painful vertebrae with extensive osteolysis or invasion secondary to benign or malignant tumor; and painful vertebral fracture associated with osteonecrosis. At least 95% of vertebroplasties performed in an institution should conform to one of those indications.[13]

Timing of the Procedure

The optimal time for intervention is not known. Most patients with painful vertebral fractures have an uneventful recovery with conventional medical therapy. Vertebral augmentation appears to relieve pain in fractures that are more than 1 year old,[14] although restoration of lost vertebral height is most likely with early intervention (within 10 weeks of the fracture).[15]

Vertebroplasty versus Kyphoplasty

Although kyphoplasty appears to provide greater restoration of lost vertebral height than vertebroplasty in appropriately selected patients, it has not been clearly demonstrated that height restoration is associated with improved long-term clinical outcomes. Vertebroplasty also restores lost vertebral height in some patients,[16] taking advantage of "dynamic mobility" (positional changes in the height of fractured vertebral bodies) by proper positioning of the patient during the procedure.[17] The risk of cement leak is probably less with kyphoplasty than vertebroplasty, although most cement leaks are mild and appear to have few clinical consequences. In many cases, the skill and experience of the proceduralist may have more to do with the success of the intervention than does the choice of intervention.

Contraindications

Vertebral augmentation should not be done in patients with nonpainful stable vertebral fractures, local or systemic infections, uncorrectable coagulopathy, hypersensitivity to any component intended for use, or retropulsed fracture fragment or tumor mass that may compromise the spinal canal.

Complications

The most common complication is transient pain and tenderness at the needle entry sites, sometimes with ecchymosis or hematoma. Posterior or lateral leakage of bone cement may cause spinal cord or nerve root compression. Rib fractures have been reported because of force applied to the spine with the patient in the prone position.

Summary

Vertebroplasty and kyphoplasty appear to provide rapid relief of vertebral fracture pain with a low risk of serious complications. It is uncertain whether long-term clinical outcomes are significantly different from conventional medical therapy. The benefits of restoration of lost vertebral height are unknown. More study is needed to define the optimal role of vertebral augmentation in clinical practice.

References

1. Johnell O, Kanis JA. An estimate of the worldwide prevalence and disability associated with osteoporotic fractures. Osteoporos Int. 2006;17(12):1726–33.

2. Boonen S, Wahl DA, Nauroy L, et al. Balloon kyphoplasty and vertebroplasty in the management of vertebral compression fractures. Osteoporos Int. 2011;22(12):2915–34.

3. Lewiecki EM. Vertebroplasty and kyphoplasty update. Curr Osteoporos Rep. 2008;6(3):114–19.

4. Lindsay R, Silverman SL, Cooper C, et al. Risk of new vertebral fracture in the year following a fracture. JAMA. 2001;285(3):320–23.

5. National Osteoporosis Foundation. Clinician's Guide to Prevention and Treatment of Osteoporosis. National Osteoporosis Foundation [Electronic version]. Available: http://www.nof.org/sites/default/files/pdfs/NOF_ClinicianGuide2009_v7.pdf. Accessibility verified March 21, 2012.

6. Buchbinder R, Osborne RH, Ebeling PR, et al. A randomized trial of vertebroplasty for painful osteoporotic vertebral fractures. N Engl J Med. 2009;361(6):557–68.

7. Kallmes DF, Comstock BA, Heagerty PJ, et al. A randomized trial of vertebroplasty for osteoporotic spinal fractures. N Engl J Med. 2009;361(6):569–79.

8. Wardlaw D, Cummings SR, Van Meirhaeghe J, et al. Efficacy and safety of balloon kyphoplasty compared with non-surgical care for vertebral compression fracture (FREE): a randomised controlled trial. Lancet. 2009;373(9668):1016–24.

9. Boonen S, Van Meirhaeghe J, Bastian L, et al. Balloon kyphoplasty for the treatment of acute vertebral compression fractures: 2-year results from a randomized trial. J Bone Miner Res. 2011;26(7):1627–37.

10. Rotter R, Martin H, Fuerderer S, et al. Vertebral body stenting: a new method for vertebral augmentation versus kyphoplasty. Eur Spine J. 2010;19(6):916–23.

11. Klezl Z, Majeed H, Bommireddy R, et al. Early results after vertebral body stenting for fractures of the anterior column of the thoracolumbar spine. Injury. 2011;42(10):1038–42.

12. Fink A, Kosecoff J, Chassin M, et al. Consensus methods: characteristics and guidelines for use. Am J Public Health. 1984;74(9):979–83.

13. McGraw JK, Cardella J, Barr JD, et al. Society of Interventional Radiology quality improvement guidelines for percutaneous vertebroplasty. J Vasc Interv Radiol. 2003;14(7):827–31.

14. Kaufmann TJ, Jensen ME, Schweickert PA, et al. Age of fracture and clinical outcomes of percutaneous vertebroplasty. AJNR Am J Neuroradiol. 2001;22(10):1860–63.

15. Crandall D, Slaughter D, Hankins PJ, et al. Acute versus chronic vertebral compression fractures treated with kyphoplasty: early results. Spine J. 2004;4(4):418–24.

16. Pitton MB, Morgen N, Herber S, et al. Height gain of vertebral bodies and stabilization of vertebral geometry over one year after vertebroplasty of osteoporotic vertebral fractures. Eur Radiol. 2008;18(3):608–15.

17. McKiernan F, Jensen R, Faciszewski T. The dynamic mobility of vertebral compression fractures. J Bone Miner Res. 2003;18(1):24–29.

Chapter 11

Glucocorticoid-Induced Osteoporosis

Glucocorticoid therapy is associated with dose-dependent bone demineraliza-tion and increased fracture risk that is partly independent of the decrease in BMD.[1] Bone loss is most pronounced during the first 3 months of therapy, peaking at about 6 months, and then continuing at a slower rate.[2] Fracture risk is related to the daily and cumulative dose.[1,2] Even small doses—2.5 mg prednisone daily[3] and inhaled glucocorticoids[4]—are associated with detrimen-tal skeletal effects. The increased risk of fractures declines when glucocorticoid administration is discontinued and is not increased in patients on glucocorticoid replacement therapy for adrenal insufficiency.[1]

Mechanisms of Glucocorticoid-Induced Bone Demineralization and Increased Fracture Risk

Several factors contribute to bone loss and fractures associated with gluco-corticoid therapy,[5,6] including osteoblastic inhibition: replication, differentia-tion, maturation, and increased apoptosis; osteoclastic stimulation: increased expression of receptor activator of nuclear factor kappa-B ligand (RANKL), decreased osteoprotegerin expression (see Chapter 2) and decreased apop-tosis; impaired osteocyte function and increased apoptosis; reduced gastroin-testinal calcium absorption; increased renal calcium excretion; reduced gonadal hormones; myopathy, muscle atrophy, and impaired neuromuscular functions; impaired bone strength; and increased bone fragility.

Assessing Fracture Risk

Vertebral fracture assessment (VFA) identifies patients who have already sus-tained vertebral fractures and therefore are at risk of further fractures.[7] The FRAX® tool, although useful to estimate the fracture risk, overestimates the risk in patients on less than prednisone 2.5 mg daily and underestimates it in patients on more than 7.5 mg daily.[1] The American College of Rheumatology developed an easy-to-use nomogram to estimate the fracture risk of patients on glucocor-ticoids based on the patient's gender, ethnic group, and T-score. Patients are classified into high-, medium-, and low-risk groups.[2] The following factors may shift the patient's risk to a higher category: low body mass index, parental history of hip fracture, current cigarette smoking, three or more daily alcoholic drinks, high daily or cumulative dose of glucocorticoids, intravenous glucocorticoids, and decreasing BMD.[2] Assessing the risk of falls and fractures may be indicated in some patients. Several tools are available (Figs. 11.1 and 11.2).[8]

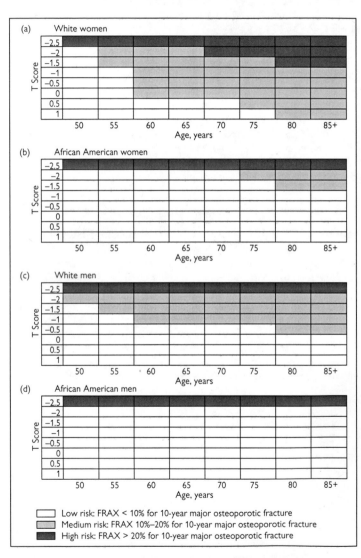

Figure 11.1 American College of Rheumatology Fracture Risk Stratification.

Reprinted with permission from Grossman JM, Gordon R, Ranganath VK, et al. American College of Rheumatology 2010 recommendations for the prevention and treatment of glucocorticoid-induced osteoporosis. Arthritis Care Res (Hoboken). 2010;62(11):1515–26.

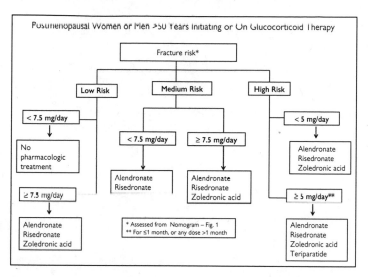

Figure 11.2 Fracture risk for Postmenopausal Women or Men More Than 50 Years Initiating or on Glucocorticoid Therapy.

Adapted and reprinted with permission from Grossman JM, Gordon R, Ranganath VK, et al. American College of Rheumatology 2010 recommendations for the prevention and treatment of glucocorticoid-induced osteoporosis. Arthritis Care Res (Hoboken). 2010;62(11):1515–26.

Management of Glucocorticoid-Induced Osteoporosis

In addition to using the smallest effective dose for the shortest period, several avenues are available to reduce the negative impact of glucocorticoids on bone mass. Although algorithms are available to guide clinicians to best manage patients on glucocorticoids,[2,9] the ultimate decisions should be modulated by the clinician's experience and the individual circumstances of the patient.

1. ***General measures:*** The patient must get an adequate daily amount of calcium and vitamin D. Because glucocorticoids increase renal calcium loss and interfere with the absorption of calcium through the gastrointestinal tract, the daily intake of calcium should be higher than the recommended allowance.[10]

2. ***Bone demineralization:*** Identify and manage other causes of bone demineralization, especially hypovitaminosis D.

3. ***Antiresorptives:*** Several studies have documented the usefulness of antiresorptives in the management of glucocorticoid-induced osteoporosis, including alendronate,[11] risedronate,[12] ibandronate,[13] zoledronic acid,[14] raloxifene,[15] and calcitonin.[16]

4. ***Osteoanabolics:*** teriparatide.[17] There is no indication that combining an antiresorptive with an osteoanabolic improves outcome.[18]

5. ***Hydrochlorothiazide:*** In small doses (12.5 mg daily) may reduce renal calcium loss. Such low doses are not usually sufficient to impact blood

pressure, induce orthostatic hypotension, aggravate diabetes mellitus, or lead to negative metabolic complications such as hyperuricemia and hypercholesterolemia.

Patient Monitoring

Monitoring includes height, BMD, and serum vitamin D measurements, incidence of fragility fractures, and compliance with prescribed medication.[2]

References

1. Leib ES, Saag KG, Adachi JD, et al. Official Positions for FRAX(®) clinical regarding glucocorticoids: the impact of the use of glucocorticoids on the estimate by FRAX(®) of the 10 year risk of fracture from Joint Official Positions Development Conference of the International Society for Clinical Densitometry and International Osteoporosis Foundation on FRAX(®). J Clin Densitom. 2011;14(3):212–19.

2. Grossman JM, Gordon R, Ranganath VK, et al. American College of Rheumatology 2010 recommendations for the prevention and treatment of glucocorticoid-induced osteoporosis. Arthritis Care Res (Hoboken). 2010;62(11):1515–26.

3. Van Staa TP, Leufkens HG, Abenhaim L, et al. Use of oral glucocorticoids and risk of fractures. J Bone Miner Res. 2000;15(6):993–1000.

4. Israel E, Banerjee TR, Fitzmaurice GM, et al. Effects of inhaled glucocorticoids on bone density in premenopausal women. N Engl J Med. 2001;345(13):941–47.

5. Pereira RM, Carvalho JF, Canalis E. Glucocorticoid-induced osteoporosis in rheumatic diseases. Clinics (Sao Paulo). 2010;65(11):1197–205.

6. Canalis E, Mazziotti G, Giustina A, et al. Glucocorticoid-induced osteoporosis: pathophysiology and therapy. Osteoporos Int. 2007;18(10):1319–28.

7. Lewiecki EM, Laster AJ. Clinical review: clinical applications of vertebral fracture assessment by dual-energy x-ray absorptiometry. J Clin Endocrinol Metab. 2006;91(11):4215–22.

8. Ganz DA, Bao Y, Shekelle PG, et al. Will my patient fall? JAMA. 2007;297(1):77–86.

9. Compston J. Clinical question: What is the best approach to managing glucocorticoid-induced osteoporosis? Clin Endocrinol (Oxf). 2011;74(5):547–50.

10. Holick MF. Optimal vitamin D status for the prevention and treatment of osteoporosis. Drugs Aging. 2007;24(12):1017–29.

11. Prinsloo PJ, Hosking DJ. Alendronate sodium in the management of osteoporosis. Ther Clin Risk Manag. 2006;2(3):235–49.

12. Mok CC, Tong KH, To CH, et al. Risedronate for prevention of bone mineral density loss in patients receiving high-dose glucocorticoids: a randomized double-blind placebo-controlled trial. Osteoporos Int. 2008;19(3):357–64.

13. Ringe JD, Dorst A, Faber H, et al. Intermittent intravenous ibandronate injections reduce vertebral fracture risk in glucocorticoid-induced osteoporosis: results from a long-term comparative study. Osteoporos Int. 2003;14(10):801–07.

14. Reid DM, Devogelaer JP, Saag K, et al. Zoledronic acid and risedronate in the prevention and treatment of glucocorticoid-induced osteoporosis (HORIZON): a multicentre, double-blind, double-dummy, randomised controlled trial. Lancet. 2009;373(9671):1253–63.

15. Mok CC, Ying KY, To CH, et al. Raloxifene for prevention of glucocorticoid-induced bone loss: a 12-month randomised double-blinded placebo-controlled trial. Ann Rheum Dis. 2011;70(5):778–84.

16. Adachi JD, Bensen WG, Bell MJ, et al. Salmon calcitonin nasal spray in the prevention of glucocorticoid-induced osteoporosis. Br J Rheumatol. 1997;36(2):255–59.

17. Saag KG, Zanchetta JR, Devogelaer JP, et al. Effects of teriparatide versus alendronate for treating glucocorticoid-induced osteoporosis: thirty-six-month results of a randomized, double-blind, controlled trial. Arthritis Rheum. 2009;60(11):3346–55.

18. Devogelaer JP, Goemaere S, Boonen S, et al. Evidence-based guidelines for the prevention and treatment of glucocorticoid-induced osteoporosis: a consensus document of the Belgian Bone Club. Osteoporos Int. 2006;17(1):8–19.

Chapter 12

Primary Hyperparathyroidism

Background

Primary hyperparathyroidism (PHPT) is a common endocrine disorder, with an incidence as high as 1 in 500. It is about three times more common in women than men; many are diagnosed in the first decade after menopause. About 80% of patients have a single benign parathyroid adenoma, with most others having hyperplasia of all four parathyroid glands. Rarely (<0.5% of patients), parathyroid carcinoma is the cause. Skeletal complications are a consequence of PHPT, with a pattern of bone disease different than postmenopausal osteoporosis. Advanced or "classical" PHPT is characterized by long-standing parathyroid hormone (PTH) elevation with hypercalcemia, presenting clinically as generalized or focal bone pain, fragility fractures, or localized areas of bone swelling. Radiographic findings include subperiosteal resorption of distal phalanges, tapering of distal clavicles, "salt and pepper" appearance of the skull, and brown tumors of bones (focal areas of extensive bone resorption with fibrous replacement).[1] When surgically excised, these tumors are typically composed of soft friable red-brown material; histologically there is accumulation of giant cells in a fibrovascular stroma with cystic spaces and hemorrhagic foci.

With the widespread use of automated blood chemistry screening, PHPT is now typically diagnosed and treated long before overt symptoms and signs of skeletal disease occur. PHPT usually comes to clinical attention through the finding of mild hypercalcemia on routine laboratory testing in patients without well-defined skeletal symptoms or by measuring serum PTH in the course of evaluating patients with osteoporosis.

Bone Remodeling

In PHPT, the rate of bone remodeling is elevated. However, in contrast to the excess resorption over formation that occurs in women with postmenopausal osteoporosis, bone resorption and formation remain in balance.[2] Bone biopsies in patients with PHPT typically show a reduction in cortical width and an increase in cortical porosity, with preservation or enhancement of trabecular bone structure. On the other hand, women with postmenopausal osteoporosis have a reduction in trabecular volume as well as a decrease in cortical thickness. The beneficial effect of PTH on trabecular bone in postmenopausal women with mild PHPT in part may result from prolongation of the active bone formation phase in individual remodeling units.[3]

Bone Density

The pattern of bone loss in PHPT is strikingly different than in postmenopausal osteoporosis. Bone loss with postmenopausal osteoporosis is greatest at skeletal sites with a large trabecular component, with bone mineral density (BMD) being lowest in the lumbar spine, relatively well-preserved in the one-third radius, and intermediate at the hip. With PHPT, the pattern is reversed, with BMD often lowest at the one-third radius, preservation at the lumbar spine, and intermediate at the hip.[4,5] These findings are consistent with chronic elevation of PTH having a catabolic effect on cortical bone and an anabolic effect on trabecular bone. A portion of the observed reduction in BMD at the radius may be an artifact of increased bone diameter, leading to a decrease in areal BMD measured by dual-energy x-ray absorptiometry (DXA).[6]

Fracture Risk

It is not clear whether the relationship between BMD and fracture risk in men and women with PHPT is the same as for patients without PHPT. A reduction in bone strength is likely to occur with cortical thinning and increased cortical porosity in patients with PHPT, although this may be counterbalanced, at least in part, by an increase in bone diameter associated with endosteal resorption and periosteal apposition.[7]

Most studies have shown an increased risk of fractures in the spine and other skeletal sites with PHPT.[8] When 150 consecutive postmenopausal women diagnosed with PHPT were compared with 300 healthy controls, there was about a six-fold increase in prevalent vertebral fractures with PHPT.[9] In contrast, one study reported no increase in vertebral fracture risk with PHPT,[10] and another study of 674 patients with PHPT showed an increased fracture risk at some skeletal sites (e.g., spine, ankles, forearm) but not in the femoral neck,[11] with no change in fracture risk after parathyroid surgery. Considering the complexity of skeletal effects of chronic exposure to elevated PTH levels and methodologic differences in studies evaluating fracture risk, well-designed long-term studies are needed to provide a better understanding of fracture risk with PHPT and the potential alteration of fracture risk with medical or surgical therapy.[12] At present, the best available evidence suggests that PHPT is associated with an increase in fracture risk at trabecular and cortical skeletal sites.

Normocalcemic Primary Hyperparathyroidism

In normocalcemic PHPT, the serum PTH is elevated, but the serum calcium and serum 25-hydroxy-vitamin D are normal. For this diagnosis to be made, potential secondary causes of PTH elevation must be ruled out, including vitamin D deficiency, chronic kidney disease, renal hypercalciuria, and malabsorption. Although data on the pathophysiology and natural history of confirmed normocalcemic PHPT are limited, the largest prospective study of these patients reported that 40% developed signs of progressive disease, including

Assessment	Indication for Parathyroidectomy
Serum calcium	>1.0 mg/dL (0.25 nmol/L) above upper limit of normal, or
Calculated creatinine clearance	<60 mL/min, or
Bone mineral density	T-score ≤–2.5 in peri- or postmenopausal women and men age 50 years and older, or Z-score ≤–2.5 in premenopausal women and men under age 50 years, or
Fracture	Previous fragility fracture, or
Age	<50 years
Symptoms	Examples: fractures, kidney stones, possibly neuromuscular or neuropsychiatric dysfunction, possibly cardiovascular disease

Figure 12.1 Indications for Parathyroid Surgery in Patients with Asymptomatic Primary Hyperparathyroidism. Surgery should be considered when any one of the included conditions is present. There are no guidelines for surgery in patients with normocalcemic primary hyperthyroidism.

Source: Bilezikian JP, Khan AA, Potts JT Jr. Guidelines for the management of asymptomatic primary hyperparathyroidism: summary statement from the third international workshop. J Clin Endocrinol Metab. 2009;94(2):335–39.

hypercalcemia, renal calculi, fractures, marked hypercalciuria, or a more than 10% decline in BMD, suggesting that this may be the earliest phase of symptomatic PHPT.[13] For most patients with normocalcemic PHPT, periodic monitoring is probably the best clinical strategy, with consideration of surgical intervention according to current guidelines for PHPT (Fig. 12.1).

Differential Diagnosis of Hypercalcemia

A patient with a serum calcium level that is persistently or intermittently elevated and an elevated or high normal (i.e. inappropriately elevated) PTH level is likely to have PHPT. The measured total serum calcium should be adjusted for serum albumin when appropriate, and in patients with acid-base disturbances, measurement of ionized serum calcium may be helpful. More than 90% of patients with hypercalcemia have either PHPT or hypercalcemia of malignancy. Familial hypocalciuric hypercalcemia (FHH), a disorder caused by inactivating mutations of calcium-sensing receptors, may cause hypercalcemia with normal or slightly elevated PTH. It is important to distinguish FHH from PHPT, because FHH is a benign condition that does not respond to parathyroidectomy. FHH is characterized by low urinary calcium excretion. When FHH is suspected, a 24-hour urine for calcium and creatinine is helpful. If the urinary calcium is less than 100 mg/24 hours or the calcium:creatinine clearance ratio ([24-hour urine calcium × serum creatinine] / [serum calcium × 24-hour urine creatinine]) is less than 0.01, it is likely that the patient has FHH. A urinary calcium level greater than 200 mg/24 hours or calcium/creatinine clearance ratio greater than 0.02 is consistent with PHPT.

Parathyroidectomy

Patients with symptomatic parathyroid disease should be referred for surgery. Symptoms of PHPT include fractures, renal calculi, and possibly neuropsychiatric dysfunction with reduced quality of life. Surgery should be performed by an experienced surgeon with the necessary resources to optimize clinical outcomes. Although preoperative imaging (e.g., ultrasonography, technetium-99m sestamibi scan, computed tomography, magnetic resonance imaging) can assist the surgeon in localizing abnormal parathyroid glands(s), negative imaging findings do not exclude the diagnosis of PHPT.

Indications for parathyroidectomy in patients with asymptomatic PHPT were developed at the Third International Workshop on the Management of Asymptomatic Hyperparathyroidism.[14] Successful parathyroid surgery is usually followed by resolution of all biochemical abnormalities, improved BMD, and reduction in fracture risk.

Nonsurgical Care

Patients who refuse surgery or are not good surgical candidates should be monitored with annual measurement of serum calcium and creatinine, plus BMD testing at three skeletal sites (lumbar spine, hip, and distal one-third radius) every 1 to 2 years.[14] Treatment involves maintaining a healthy lifestyle, avoiding drugs known to cause hypercalcemia, correcting modifiable risk factors for bone loss and fracture, and consideration of antiresorptive therapy. Restriction of dietary calcium and vitamin D intake is not advisable, because doing so may add a component of secondary hyperparathyroidism to PHPT. A daily calcium intake (diet plus supplements, if needed) of about 1,200 mg and vitamin D intake to maintain a serum 25-OH-D level of at least 20 ng/mL (50 nmol/L) is recommended.[14]

Pharmacologic Therapy

Antiresorptive agents, such as bisphosphonates and estrogen, may provide skeletal protection in patients with PHPT who are unwilling or unable to undergo parathyroid surgery.[12] Alendronate significantly increased BMD at the lumbar spine and total hip, but not the distal one-third radius, as early as 1 year compared with the baseline in patients with PHPT.[15] Women with mild PHPT taking estrogen had significantly higher BMD than controls at the lumbar spine, femoral neck, mid-radius, and distal radius.[16] Concern regarding long-term risks of estrogen has limited its use beyond relief of menopausal symptoms. In an 8-week study of raloxifene in 18 postmenopausal women with PHPT, reductions in serum calcium and BTM were observed; BMD measurements were not done.[17] In a meta-analysis of studies of patients with mild PHPT treated with no intervention, surgery, or medical therapy, BMD increased at similar rates with surgery, bisphosphonates, and hormone replacement therapy, with the magnitude of BMD increase greatest at the lumbar spine, least at the forearm, and intermediate at the femoral neck.[18]

Calcimimetics such as cinacalcet increase the sensitivity of calcium-sensing receptors of parathyroid cells and are indicated for severe hypercalcemia in patients with PHPT who are unable to undergo parathyroidectomy. Cinacalcet is also indicated for hypercalcemia in patients with parathyroid carcinoma, and for secondary hyperparathyroidism in patients with chronic kidney disease on dialysis. In a 1-year study in 78 patients with PHPT randomized to receive placebo or oral cinacalcet, those treated with cinacalcet had a rapid and sustained normalization of serum calcium and modest reduction in serum PTH, with no change in BMD.[19]

Summary

PHPT is associated with elevated bone turnover, reduction in BMD, and probably increased fracture risk. BMD loss is most pronounced at predominantly cortical bone sites, and relatively preserved at predominantly trabecular bone sites. Parathyroidectomy, the definitive treatment for PHPT, results in reduction of bone turnover, increased BMD, decreased fracture risk, and resolution of biochemical abnormalities. Bisphosphonates and estrogen appear to provide skeletal benefit similar to parathyroid surgery. The skeletal effects of raloxifene in PHPT are unclear because of lack of data. Cinacalcet may be useful in controlling intractable hypercalcemia in some patients with PHPT.

References

1. Triantafillidou K, Zouloumis L, Karakinaris G, Kalimeras E, Iordanidis F. Brown tumors of the jaws associated with primary or secondary hyperparathyroidism. A clinical study and review of the literature. Am J Otolaryngol. 2006;27(4):281–86.

2. Valdemarsson S, Lindergard B, Tibblin S, Bergenfelz A. Increased biochemical markers of bone formation and resorption in primary hyperparathyroidism with special reference to patients with mild disease. J Intern Med. 1998;243(2):115–22.

3. Dempster DW, Parisien M, Silverberg SJ, et al. On the mechanism of cancellous bone preservation in postmenopausal women with mild primary hyperparathyroidism. J Clin Endocrinol Metab. 1999;84(5):1562–66.

4. Silverberg SJ, Shane E, de la Cruz L, et al. Skeletal disease in primary hyperparathyroidism. J Bone Miner Res. 1989;4(3):283–91.

5. Parisien M, Cosman F, Mellish RW, et al. Bone structure in postmenopausal hyperparathyroid, osteoporotic, and normal women. J Bone Miner Res. 1995;10(9):1393–99.

6. Miller PD, Bilezikian JP. Bone densitometry in asymptomatic primary hyperparathyroidism. J Bone Miner Res. 2002;17 Suppl 2:N98–102.

7. Parfitt AM. Parathyroid hormone and periosteal bone expansion. J Bone Miner Res. 2002;17(10):1741–43.

8. Khosla S, Melton LJ 3rd, Wermers RA, et al. Primary hyperparathyroidism and the risk of fracture: a population-based study. J Bone Miner Res. 1999;14(10):1700–07.

9. Vignali E, Viccica G, Diacinti D, et al. Morphometric vertebral fractures in postmenopausal women with primary hyperparathyroidism. J Clin Endocrinol Metab. 2009;94(7):2306–12.

10. Wilson RJ, Rao S, Ellis B, et al. Mild asymptomatic primary hyperparathyroidism is not a risk factor for vertebral fractures. Ann Intern Med. 1988;109(12):959–62.

11. Vestergaard P, Mollerup CL, Frøkjaer VG, et al. Cohort study of risk of fracture before and after surgery for primary hyperparathyroidism. BMJ. 2000;321(7261):598–602.

12. Lewiecki EM. Management of skeletal health in patients with asymptomatic primary hyperparathyroidism. J Clin Densitom. 2010;13(4):324–34.

13. Lowe H, McMahon DJ, Rubin MR, et al. Normocalcemic primary hyperparathyroidism: further characterization of a new clinical phenotype. J Clin Endocrinol Metab. 2007;92(8):3001–05.

14. Bilezikian JP, Khan AA, Potts JT Jr. Guidelines for the management of asymptomatic primary hyperparathyroidism: summary statement from the third international workshop. J Clin Endocrinol Metab. 2009;94(2):335–39.

15. Khan AA, Bilezikian JP, Kung AW, et al. Alendronate in primary hyperparathyroidism: a double-blind, randomized, placebo-controlled trial. J Clin Endocrinol Metab. 2004;89(7):3319–25.

16. McDermott MT, Perloff JJ, Kidd GS. Effects of mild asymptomatic primary hyperparathyroidism on bone mass in women with and without estrogen replacement therapy. J Bone Miner Res. 1994;9(4):509–14.

17. Rubin MR, Lee KH, McMahon DJ, et al. Raloxifene lowers serum calcium and markers of bone turnover in postmenopausal women with primary hyperparathyroidism. J Clin Endocrinol Metab. 2003;88(3):1174–78.

18. Sankaran S, Gamble G, Bolland M, et al. Skeletal effects of interventions in mild primary hyperparathyroidism: a meta-analysis. J Clin Endocrinol Metab. 2010;95(4):1653–62.

19. Peacock M, Bilezikian JP, Klassen PS, et al. Cinacalcet hydrochloride maintains long-term normocalcemia in patients with primary hyperparathyroidism. J Clin Endocrinol Metab. 2005;90(1):135–41.

Chapter 13

Premenopausal Women

Low bone mineral density (BMD) and fractures are uncommon in premenopausal women[1] and BMD testing in premenopausal women is rarely indicated. However, when a premenopausal woman has a low trauma fracture or a disease or condition associated with low bone mass, the International Society for Clinical Densitometry (ISCD) recommends BMD testing, with the caveat that interpretation of the findings is different than in postmenopausal women.[2] It is the ISCD position that Z-scores (the standard deviation [SD] difference between the patient's BMD and the mean BMD of an age-, sex-, and ethnicity-matched reference population), not T-scores (the SD difference between the patient's BMD and the mean BMD of a young-adult sex-matched reference population), be used in expressing bone density in premenopausal women. The ISCD advises that the World Health Organization classification of osteoporosis, osteopenia, and normal according to T-score not be used in premenopausal women. In a premenopausal woman (and man under the age of 50), a Z-score of –2.0 or less is defined as "below the expected range for age" and a Z-score greater than –2.0 is defined as "within the expected range for age." These distinctions in diagnostic classification according to menstrual status in women have been made because many premenopausal women with low BMD do not have a disease (osteoporosis) associated with high fracture risk and are not likely to benefit from pharmacologic therapy intended to reduce fracture risk.[3] Many healthy premenopausal women with low BMD have low peak bone mass[4] or small bone size,[5] yet typically have normal bone structure and strength without elevation of fracture risk.

Some premenopausal women may experience low trauma fractures because of impaired bone strength caused by the same secondary factors that occur in postmenopausal women (e.g., glucocorticoids, malabsorption, hyperparathyroidism). When premenopausal women sustain fragility fractures and no secondary causes are detected, patients are classified as having idiopathic premenopausal osteoporosis. These patients have been found to have deterioration of trabecular microarchitecture as measured by high resolution peripheral computed tomography (HR-pQCT)[6] and evidence of low bone formation on iliac crest bone biopsies consistent with osteoblast dysfunction.[7]

The treatment of premenopausal women with skeletal fragility is principally directed to correction, when possible, of the underlying cause. Patients found to have celiac disease, for example, require strict lifelong adherence to a gluten-free diet, which may result in large increases in BMD and reduction in markers of bone turnover.[8] Patients with anticonvulsant bone disease may have severe vitamin D deficiency, sometimes with osteomalacia, necessitating treatment with pharmacologic doses of vitamin D. Pharmacologic intervention with agents used to treat postmenopausal women with osteoporosis should be used with caution, if at all, in premenopausal women, with careful consideration of the balance between expected benefits and potential risks. Data on efficacy and safety of these drugs in premenopausal women are limited, and there is particular concern with regard to potential adverse effects on fetal development if a treated woman of child-bearing potential becomes pregnant. Parenteral bisphosphonate therapy has been shown to benefit children and adolescents with osteogenesis imperfecta, thereby allowing them to enter adulthood with improved peak bone mass.[9]

Eating disorders, which may occur in women or men of any age, are particularly prevalent in premenopausal women and adolescent girls,[10] and may cause endocrine complications that result in bone loss and fractures.[11] Eating disorders may be categorized as anorexia nervosa, bulimia nervosa, and "not otherwise specified," which includes disordered eating behavior and weight management habits that do not meet established criteria for the diagnosis of anorexia nervosa or bulimia nervosa.

Female Athlete Triad

Female athlete triad was first defined in 1992 and introduced in the scientific literature in 1997 in a Position Stand of the American College of Sports Medicine (ACSM).[12] The triad was defined as disordered eating, amenorrhea, and osteoporosis, recognizing that not all patients have all three components of the triad, with variable manifestations of the components over time. In 2007, the ACSM published an updated definition of female athlete triad, viewing each component of the triad as a spectrum of symptoms and behaviors ranging from health to disease.[13] In this definition, "disordered eating," which has an estimated prevalence as high as 62% in female athletes,[14] is replaced by "energy availability" (with or without disordered eating), ranging from optimal to low; "amenorrhea" is replaced by "menstrual function," ranging from eumenorrhea to functional hypothalamic amenorrhea; and "osteoporosis" is replaced by "bone mineral density," ranging from optimal to osteoporosis.

A woman with female athlete triad may be healthy or may have significant health risks with potentially irreversible consequences. Low energy availability may occur when dietary intake is intentionally or inadvertently restricted, often when energy expenditure is very high, resulting in a cascade of physiologic and neuroendocrine adaptations. High levels of exercise and low body weight do not in themselves cause amenorrhea, but rather it is caused by hormonal changes resulting from low energy availability. These changes include a decrease in the frequency and amplitude of pulses of gonadotropin-releasing hormone (GnRH) in the hypothalamus, resulting in a decrease in pulsatile pituitary release of luteinizing hormone (LH) and follicle stimulating hormone (FSH), with subsequent reduction in ovarian production of estrogen and progesterone.[11] Other hormones that potentially play a role in the pathogenesis of amenorrhea include leptin, cortisol, insulin, growth hormone, and insulin-like growth factor 1 (IGF-1).

Low BMD in women with female athlete triad is probably multifactorial in origin, with failure to achieve optimal peak bone mass and/or bone loss resulting from estrogen deficiency and other hormonal disturbances. The ACSM reported a prevalence of 22% to 50% for a T-score between −1.0 and −2.5 and a prevalence of 0% to 13% for a T-score less than −2.5 in female athletes (data acquired before the ISCD recommendation to use Z-scores was released).[13] Patients with female athlete triad and low BMD are at risk for fractures, particularly stress fractures, with fracture incidence that varies according to the severity to the disease and the sport.[15] The ACSM has defined low BMD as a Z-score between −1.0 and −2.0, and osteoporosis as a Z-score of −2.0 or less in premenopausal women or girls with a history of nutritional deficiencies, low estrogen, stress fractures, and/or other secondary clinical risk factors for fracture.[13]

The treatment of female athlete triad is multidisciplinary, and may include physicians, dieticians, mental health professionals, coaches, and parents. Education of all stakeholders is an important part of the recovery process. Efforts should be undertaken to increase energy availability (improved nutrition, reduced level of training) so as to restore menstruation, and optimize BMD with nonpharmacologic therapy, with particular attention to adequacy of calcium and vitamin D intake. No pharmacologic therapy has been shown to fully restore BMD. Oral contraceptives may initiate menstrual cycles, but do not normalize the metabolic factors that are detrimental to skeletal health. The ACSM recommends consideration of oral contraceptives to prevent further loss of BMD in female athletes age 16 years or older with functional hypothalamic amenorrhea if BMD is decreasing despite adequate nutrition and body weight.[13] Bisphosphonates should not be used in these patients.

Anorexia Nervosa

Anorexia nervosa is an eating disorder characterized by abnormally low body weight, intense fear of gaining weight, distorted perception of body weight and shape, and amenorrhea. The prevalence of anorexia nervosa in young females is estimated to be about 0.3%,[16] with a peak onset between the ages of 15 and 19 years.[17] The origins of eating disorders include genetic, biologic, environmental, and social factors, sometimes associated with precipitating psychological trauma in a predisposed individual. Often there is a past history of dieting, childhood preoccupation with body weight, social pressures concerning body weight, and involvement with sports and activities (e.g., gymnastics, long distance running, ballet) that emphasize low body weight. Psychiatric problems, including affective disorders, anxiety disorders, personality disorders, and obsessive-compulsive behavior, are common. The diagnosis of anorexia nervosa should be considered when there is a failure to achieve expected growth, body mass index less than 17.5 to 18.5 kg/m^2, or weight less than 85% of ideal body weight.[18] In a meta-analysis of 36 studies with 166,642 person-years of observation, anorexia nervosa was associated with an increased mortality rate, including death by suicide.[19]

Among the numerous reported medical complications of anorexia nervosa (e.g., cardiovascular disease, infertility, gastroparesis, impaired liver function) are low BMD and increased risk of fractures.[20] Anorexia nervosa is a risk factor for reduced accrual of bone mass in adolescents and loss of bone in adults. A study of BMD in 60 adolescent girls (mean age 16 years) with anorexia nervosa found that 50% had lumbar spine Z-scores less than −1.0 and 9.1% were less than −2.0.[21] In a prospective cohort analysis of 130 women (mean age 24 years) with anorexia nervosa, 92% were reported to have a T-score less than or equal to −1.0 and 38% had a T-score less than or equal to −2.5.[22] Fracture risk was evaluated in 2,149 patients with anorexia nervosa (mean age at diagnosis 21 years), 94% of whom were female.[23] Compared with age- and gender-matched controls, fracture risk was elevated in patients with anorexia nervosa (incidence rate ratio 1.98, 95% CI 1.60–2.44). The increase in fracture risk was not observed before the diagnosis of anorexia was made, but persisted for many years after the diagnosis.[23] This is consistent with a Mayo Clinic population-based cohort study that included 193 women with anorexia nervosa.[24] Compared with expected numbers of fractures in standardized incidence ratios (SIRs), fracture risk was increased with anorexia nervosa (SIR 2.9, 95% CI 1.1–7.9), with the increased risk persisting later in life.

HR-pQCT has been used to assess bone quality in patients with anorexia nervosa. Adolescent girls and adult women with this disorder have reduced trabecular bone volume, reduced trabecular thickness, and greater trabecular separation than controls.[25] Finite element analysis documents reduced bone strength parameters in patients with anorexia nervosa compared with controls. There are many factors that contribute to low BMD and high fracture risk with anorexia nervosa. Abnormalities of bone remodeling has been reported, with uncoupling of remodeling (increase in bone resorption markers and decrease in bone formation markers) in adults and reduced rate of remodeling (low levels of bone resorption and formation markers) in adolescents with anorexia nervosa.[25] The magnitude of bone loss appears to be associated with body mass index, lean body mass, and duration of amenorrhea. Numerous hormonal abnormalities seen with anorexia nervosa are associated with adverse skeletal effects, including low serum levels of estrogen, androgens, IGF-1, and leptin, elevated serum cortisol, and growth hormone resistance.[25]

The best established treatment for low BMD in premenopausal women with anorexia nervosa is weight gain with resumption of menstrual function and resolution of hormonal abnormalities. All patients should receive an adequate daily intake of calcium and vitamin D in addition to other essential nutrients. Most studies have shown no beneficial effect of oral contraceptives or estrogen in improving bone mass in premenopausal women. There is limited evidence that treatment with IGF-1 may be effective, but more study is needed before this can be recommended for use in clinical practice. The use of bisphosphonates in premenopausal women is discouraged because of unproven efficacy and safety concerns regarding potential adverse effects on fetal skeletal development in the case of subsequent pregnancy.

References

1. Thompson PW, Taylor J, Dawson A. The annual incidence and seasonal variation of fractures of the distal radius in men and women over 25 years in Dorset, UK. Injury. 2004;35(5):462–66.

2. Baim S, Binkley N, Bilezikian JP, et al. Official Positions of the International Society for Clinical Densitometry and executive summary of the 2007 ISCD Position Development Conference. J Clin Densitom. 2008;11:75–91.

3. Lewiecki EM. Premenopausal bone health assessment. Curr Rheumatol Rep. 2005;7(1):46–52.

4. Heaney RP, Abrams S, Dawson-Hughes B, et al. Peak bone mass. Osteoporos Int. 2000;11(12):985–1009.

5. Katzman DK, Bachrach LK, Carter DR, et al. Clinical and anthropometric correlates of bone mineral acquisition in healthy adolescent girls. J Clin Endocrinol Metab. 1991;73(6):1332–39.

6. Cohen A, Liu XS, Stein EM, et al. Bone microarchitecture and stiffness in premenopausal women with idiopathic osteoporosis. J Clin Endocrinol Metab. 2009;94(11):4351–60.

7. Donovan MA, Dempster D, Zhou H, et al. Low bone formation in premenopausal women with idiopathic osteoporosis. J Clin Endocrinol Metab. 2005;90(6):3331–36.

8. Sategna-Guidetti C, Grosso SB, Grosso S, et al. The effects of 1-year gluten withdrawal on bone mass, bone metabolism and nutritional status in newly-diagnosed adult coeliac disease patients. Aliment Pharmacol Ther. 2000;14(1):35–43.

9. Rauch F, Plotkin H, Zeitlin L, et al. Bone mass, size, and density in children and adolescents with osteogenesis imperfecta: effect of intravenous pamidronate therapy. J Bone Miner Res. 2003;18(4):610–14.

10. Dalle Grave R. Eating disorders: progress and challenges. Eur J Intern Med. 2011;22(2):153–60.

11. Warren MP. Endocrine manifestations of eating disorders. J Clin Endocrinol Metab. 2011;96(2):333–43.

12. Otis CL, Drinkwater B, Johnson M, et al. American College of Sports Medicine position stand. The Female Athlete Triad. Med Sci Sports Exerc. 1997;29(5):i-ix.

13. Nattiv A, Loucks AB, Manore MM, et al. American College of Sports Medicine position stand. The female athlete triad. Med Sci Sports Exerc. 2007;39(10):1867–82.

14. Bonci CM, Bonci LJ, Granger LR, et al. National athletic trainers' association position statement: preventing, detecting, and managing disordered eating in athletes. J Athl Train. 2008;43(1):80–108.

15. Feingold D, Hame SL. Female athlete triad and stress fractures. Orthop Clin North Am. 2006;37(4):575–83.

16. Hoek HW, van Hoeken D. Review of the prevalence and incidence of eating disorders. Int J Eat Disord. 2003;34(4):383–96.

17. Lucas AR, Beard CM, O'Fallon WM, et al. Anorexia nervosa in Rochester, Minnesota: a 45-year study. Mayo Clin Proc. 1988;63(5):433–42.

18. Bulik CM, Reba L, Siega-Riz AM, et al. Anorexia nervosa: definition, epidemiology, and cycle of risk. Int J Eat Disord. 2005;37 Suppl.S2–9.

19. Arcelus J, Mitchell AJ, Wales J, et al. Mortality rates in patients with anorexia nervosa and other eating disorders. A meta-analysis of 36 studies. Arch Gen Psychiatry. 2011;68(7):724–31.

20. Misra M, Klibanski A. Bone health in anorexia nervosa. Curr Opin Endocrinol Diabetes Obes. 2011;18(6):376–82.

21. Misra M, Aggarwal A, Miller KK, et al. Effects of anorexia nervosa on clinical, hematologic, biochemical, and bone density parameters in community-dwelling adolescent girls. Pediatrics. 2004;114(6):1574–83.

22. Grinspoon S, Thomas E, Pitts S, et al. Prevalence and predictive factors for regional osteopenia in women with anorexia nervosa. Ann Intern Med. 2000;133(10):790–94.

23. Vestergaard P, Emborg C, Støving RK, et al. Fractures in patients with anorexia nervosa, bulimia nervosa, and other eating disorders--a nationwide register study. Int J Eat Disord. 2002;32(3):301–08.

24. Lucas AR, Melton LJ 3rd, Crowson CS, et al. Long-term fracture risk among women with anorexia nervosa: a population-based cohort study. Mayo Clin Proc. 1999;74(10):972–77.

25. Misra M, Klibanski A. The neuroendocrine basis of anorexia nervosa and its impact on bone metabolism. Neuroendocrinology. 2011;93(2):65–73.

26. Franco KN. Eating Disorders. Cleveland Clinic [Electronic version]. Available at: http://www.clevelandclinicmeded.com/medicalpubs/diseasemanagement/psychiatry-psychology/eating-disorders/#s0015. Accessibility verified March 21, 2012.

Chapter 14

Men

Osteoporosis is a major public health problem in older men. In a study of men age 60 years and older, the mortality-adjusted lifetime risk of fracture was 25%, and among those with a T-score of −2.5 or less, the risk increased to 42%.[1] Although osteoporotic fractures occur about 5 to 10 years later in life in men than in women, men account for approximately 30% of hip fractures and 20% of symptomatic vertebral fractures.[2] The age-adjusted mortality after a hip fracture and other types of osteoporotic fractures is higher in men than in women.[3] Despite what is known about the prevalence and serious consequences of osteoporosis in men, they are under-represented in referrals for bone density testing, underdiagnosed, and undertreated.[4,5]

Pathogenesis

Osteoporosis in men is categorized as primary (age-related), secondary (which includes the same nonhormonal factors that contribute to osteoporosis in women), and idiopathic (which may represent unrecognized secondary causes of osteoporosis). Genetic factors are important in the achievement of peak bone mass in men, with estrogen levels perhaps as important for the acquisition and maintenance of bone mass in men as in women.[6] Men lose bone mass with age, without the accelerated decline in BMD that women experience around the time of menopause. Contributors to age-related bone loss in men include poor calcium intake, lack of exercise, changes in bone remodeling, and declining sex steroid levels. In a cohort of 2,623 men older than age 65 years in the Osteoporotic Fractures in Men Study (MrOS), a significant decline in serum free testosterone and free estradiol was observed in association with an increase in serum sex hormone binding globulin (SHBG).[7] Decreases in bioavailable testosterone and bioavailable estrogen both appear to play a role in the pathogenesis of age-related bone loss and fracture risk in men, with accumulating evidence that estrogen may be the dominant factor.[8] In the Swedish arm of MrOS, multivariate proportional hazards regression models showed that free estradiol and SHBG, but not free testosterone, were independently associated with fracture risk.[9] The same study showed a threshold effect, with an increase in fracture risk in men with serum free estradiol less than 16 pg/mL.

Secondary causes have been identified in 30% to 60% of men with osteoporosis[10] with variability in prevalence according to the population studied, the extent of the evaluation, and thresholds for defining normal reference ranges. The three major secondary causes of osteoporosis in men are excessive alcohol intake, glucocorticoids (usually exogenous), and hypogonadism, which is increasingly caused by the use of androgen deprivation therapy for prostate cancer[11] Examples of other secondary causes of osteoporosis in men include hyperparathyroidism, malabsorption (e.g., celiac disease, inflammatory bowel disease, bariatric surgery), excess thyroid hormone, anticonvulsant therapy, selective serotonin reuptake inhibitors, malignancy, cigarette smoking, idiopathic hypercalciuria, and immobilization.

The use of new technologies, such as quantitative computed tomography (QCT), to measure volumetric BMD and bone structure has enhanced understanding of the pattern of age-related bone loss in men. Men, on average, have larger bones than women, accounting for higher areal BMD values measured by DXA. Because larger bones have a greater resistance to bending than smaller bones, bone size accounts, at least in part, for the lower fracture risk in men compared with women. Riggs et al. have shown both men and women have loss of volumetric BMD (measured by QCT) of trabecular bone beginning in young-adulthood, whereas cortical bone loss begins after midlife.[12] Women, however, are more likely to have loss (perforation with loss of connectivity) of trabecular structural elements, with men more likely to have trabecular thinning, as assessed by high resolution peripheral QCT (HR-pQCT) of the ultradistal radius.[13] These differences may be caused by different patterns of bone remodeling in men and women, with perimenopausal and postmenopausal women typically having an acceleration of bone remodeling with a high rate of bone resorption, whereas bone loss in men is driven by low bone formation without a high remodeling rate. Sexual dimorphism occurs with age-related changes in cortical bone as well. In aging men and women, there is endocortical bone resorption that results in cortical thinning; however, periosteal apposition, a compensatory mechanism that attenuates the deleterious effects of endocortical loss, is greater in men than in women.[14] Age-related increases in cortical porosity also appear to be less in men than in women.

Diagnosis

The International Society for Clinical Densitometry (ISCD) and the National Osteoporosis Foundation recommend BMD testing for all men age 70 years and older, regardless of clinical risk factors, and for men age 50 to 69 when risk factors are present.[15] The occurrence of a low-trauma fracture (especially at the spine or hip) or a T-score that is −2.5 or lower at the lumbar spine, femoral neck, total hip, or 33% radius in men age 50 and older is consistent with a diagnosis of osteoporosis.[16] Appropriate testing should be conducted to determine whether other causes of skeletal fragility or low BMD are present before a diagnosis of osteoporosis is confirmed. The ISCD recommends that a male reference database be used for calculation of T-scores in men in clinical practice.[16] The World Health Organization (WHO) and the International Osteoporosis Foundation, on the other hand, have established an international reference standard for the densitometric diagnosis of osteoporosis using BMD measured at the femoral neck, not other skeletal sites, with a female, not male, reference database for T-score calculation in both women and men.[17] Using a male reference database results in a lower T-score for men than when a female database is used. When diagnostic classification and treatment recommendations in men use T-score cutoffs, the selection of the reference database becomes more than a trivial matter, because it may alter the diagnosis and decision to treat There is evidence to support both options for reference databases, with no clear "correct" choice.[18]

If men and women have similar fracture rates with the same absolute BMD, then it logically follows that the same reference database should be used to calculate T-scores for both men and women. This viewpoint is supported by evidence suggesting that men and women have equivalent hip fracture risk at the same absolute hip BMD.[19] If men and women have different fracture rates with the same absolute BMD values, then it would be appropriate to use a female reference database for calculation of T-scores in women and a male reference database for calculation of T-scores in men. This is supported by evidence that men may have an increased vertebral fracture risk compared with women with the same spine BMD.[20]

Assessment of Fracture Risk

In men as well as women, there is a robust correlation between BMD and fracture risk, with fracture risk increasing as BMD decreases.[8] The WHO fracture risk assessment tool, FRAX®, can be used to estimate the 10-year probability of major osteoporotic fracture (clinical spine, forearm, hip or shoulder fracture) and the 10-year probability of hip fracture in untreated men from age 40 to 90 years.[21] FRAX®, in turn, is a component of many country-specific treatment guidelines, based on the observation that patients at high risk for fracture are most likely to benefit from pharmacologic therapy.[22]

Evaluation

All men with osteoporosis should be evaluated for factors that may contribute to skeletal fragility and possibly alter treatment choices. Some diseases, such as osteomalacia, may mimic osteoporosis yet need to be treated differently. In the presence of severe vitamin D deficiency, treatment with a potent antiresorptive agent may be ineffective and perhaps harmful, resulting in symptomatic hypocalcemia. In general, the laboratory evaluation in men is similar to women. In addition, measurement of serum testosterone may be helpful when hypogonadism is suspected. Although there is a correlation between estrogen levels and fractures in men, the clinical utility and therapeutic implications of low estrogen in men are unclear.

Treatment

The treatment of osteoporosis in men includes regular weight-bearing exercises, fall prevention, adequate daily intake of calcium and vitamin D, and avoidance of excess alcohol, cigarette smoking, and, if possible, medications known to have harmful skeletal effects. Secondary causes of osteoporosis and factors contributing to low BMD and high fracture risk should be identified and treated (see Chapters 5 and 6).

Clinical trials to evaluate the efficacy and safety of medications for the treatment of osteoporosis in men are fewer, smaller, and shorter in duration than for women. Once a drug has been proved to reduce vertebral fractures in postmenopausal women with osteoporosis and is approved for treatment in women, a smaller study in osteoporotic men with BMD as the primary endpoint may be conducted. For regulatory purposes, a similar BMD response in men is assumed to represent a similar improvement in bone strength and reduction in fracture risk. At the time of this writing , drugs approved by the US Food and Drug Administration (FDA) for the treatment of osteoporosis in men, including glucocorticoid-induced osteoporosis are: alendronate, risedronate, zoledronic acid, and teriparatide.[8] In September 2011, the FDA also approved denosumab to increase bone mass in men at high risk of fracture from receiving androgen deprivation therapy for nonmetastatic prostate cancer.[23] More recently, denosumab was approved to increase bone mass in men with osteoporosis at high risk for fracture. In men with nonmetastatic prostate cancer denosumab reduced the incidence of vertebral fracture.[23] Risedronate and zoledronic acid are also approved for the prevention of glucocorticoid-induced osteoporosis in men. Drugs approved for the treatment of men with osteoporosis appear to be equally effective in eugonadal and hypogonadal men.

Testosterone therapy improves BMD in hypogonadal men but not those with normal baseline testosterone levels.[24] The long-term safety of testosterone therapy for older men is uncertain,[25] with concern that testosterone therapy might convert an occult prostate cancer to a clinically apparent one[26] and increase the risk of adverse cardiovascular events.[27] If testosterone therapy is intended, it is reasonable to do a baseline digital rectal exam and measure the prostate specific antigen (PSA), repeat these periodically, and have a low threshold for performing a prostate biopsy.[28] Because bisphosphonate and teriparatide have been shown to be effective in both eugonadal and hypogonadal men, with a favorable balance of benefit and risk, testosterone replacement is probably best used only in men with well-established symptomatic hypogonadism.[8]

References

1. Nguyen ND, Ahlborg HG, Center JR, et al. Residual lifetime risk of fractures in women and men. J Bone Miner Res. 2007;22(6):781–88.

2. Eastell R, Boyle IT, Compston J, et al. Management of male osteoporosis: report of the UK Consensus Group. QJM. 1998;91(2):71–92.

3. Center JR, Nguyen TV, Schneider D, et al. Mortality after all major types of osteoporotic fracture in men and women: an observational study. Lancet. 1999;353(9156):878–82.

4. Kiebzak GM, Beinart GA, Perser K, et al. Undertreatment of osteoporosis in men with hip fracture. Arch Intern Med. 2002;162(19):2217–22.

5. Feldstein AC, Nichols G, Orwoll E, et al. The near absence of osteoporosis treatment in older men with fractures. Osteoporos Int. 2005;16(8):953–62.

6. Bilezikian JP, Morishima A, Bell J, et al. Increased bone mass as a result of estrogen therapy in a man with aromatase deficiency. N Engl J Med. 1998;339(9):599–603.

7. Orwoll E, Lambert LC, Marshall LM, et al. Testosterone and estradiol among older men. J Clin Endocrinol Metab. 2006;91(4):1336–44.

8. Kanis JA, Bianchi G, Bilezikian JP, et al. Towards a diagnostic and therapeutic consensus in male osteoporosis. Osteoporos Int. 2011;22(11):2789–98.

9. Mellström D, Vandenput L, Mallmin H, et al. Older men with low serum estradiol and high serum SHBG have an increased risk of fractures. J Bone Miner Res. 2008;23(10):1552–60.10. Binkley N. Osteoporosis in men. Arq Bras Endocrinol Metabol. 2006;50(4):764–74.

11. Smith MR. Treatment-related osteoporosis in men with prostate cancer. Clin Cancer Res. 2006;12(20 Pt 2):6315s-19s.

12. Riggs BL, Melton Iii LJ 3rd, Robb RA, et al. Population-based study of age and sex differences in bone volumetric density, size, geometry, and structure at different skeletal sites. J Bone Miner Res. 2004;19(12):1945–54.

13. Khosla S, Riggs BL, Atkinson EJ, et al. Effects of sex and age on bone microstructure at the ultradistal radius: a population-based noninvasive in vivo assessment. J Bone Miner Res. 2006;21(1):124–31.

14. Szulc P, Seeman E. Thinking inside and outside the envelopes of bone: dedicated to PDD. Osteoporos Int. 2009;20(8):1281–88.

15. National Osteoporosis Foundation. Clinician's Guide to Prevention and Treatment of Osteoporosis. National Osteoporosis Foundation [Electronic version]. Available: http://www.nof.org/sites/default/files/pdfs/NOF_ClinicianGuide2009_v7.pdf. Accessibility verified March 21, 2012.

16. Baim S, Binkley N, Bilezikian JP, et al. Official Positions of the International Society for Clinical Densitometry and executive summary of the 2007 ISCD Position Development Conference. J Clin Densitom. 2008;11:75–91.

17. Kanis JA, McCloskey EV, Johansson H, et al. A reference standard for the description of osteoporosis. Bone. 2008;42(3):467–75.

18. Binkley N, Lewiecki EM. The evolution of fracture risk estimation. J Bone Miner Res. 2010;25(10):2098–100.

19. De Laet CE, Van Hout BA, Burger H, et al. Hip fracture prediction in elderly men and women: validation in the Rotterdam study. J Bone Miner Res. 1998;13(10):1587–93.

20. Orwoll E. Assessing bone density in men. J Bone Miner Res. 2000;15(10):1867–70.

21. World Health Organization. FRAX WHO Fracture Risk Assessment Tool. World Health Organization [Electronic version]. Available: http://www.shef.ac.uk/FRAX/. Accessibility verified March 21, 2012.

22. Kanis JA, Oden A, Johansson H, et al. FRAX and its applications to clinical practice. Bone. 2009;44(5):734–43.

23. FDA, available at http://www.cancer.gov/cancertopics/druginfo/fda-denosumab. Last checked September 2012.

24. Snyder PJ, Peachey H, Hannoush P, et al. Effect of testosterone treatment on body composition and muscle strength in men over 65 years of age. J Clin Endocrinol Metab. 1999;84(8):2647–53.

25. Gruenewald DA, Matsumoto AM. Testosterone supplementation therapy for older men: potential benefits and risks. J Am Geriatr Soc. 2003;51(1):101–15.

26. Curran MJ, Bihrle W 3rd. Dramatic rise in prostate-specific antigen after androgen replacement in a hypogonadal man with occult adenocarcinoma of the prostate. Urology. 1999;53(2):423–24.

27. Basaria S, Coviello AD, Travison TG, et al. Adverse events associated with testosterone administration. N Engl J Med. 2010;363(2):109–22.

28. Rhoden EL, Morgentaler A. Risks of testosterone-replacement therapy and recommendations for monitoring. N Engl J Med. 2004;350(5):482–92.

Chapter 15

Osteoporosis in Children and Adolescents

In younger individuals, particularly children and adolescents (5–19 years old), the relationship between bone mineral density (BMD) and fracture risk is less well defined than in adults,[1–3] and the implications for treatment are uncertain. The International Society for Clinical Densitometry (ISCD) has recommended the use of Z-scores, not T-scores, in females before perimenopause and males less than age 50 years, defining a Z-score less than or equal to −2.0 as "below the expected range for age" and a Z-score greater than −2.0 as "within the expected range for age."[2] Yet, until recently, standards for measurement of BMD and other biomarkers of skeletal health in children and adolescents were not available, and most experts were reluctant to diagnose osteoporosis in children and adolescents without clear evidence of skeletal fragility, such as a low-trauma fracture.[4] In 2007, the ISCD convened a Position Development Conference to review the medical evidence and develop recommendations for skeletal health assessment in children and adolescents.[5] This provided guidance for clinicians and identified topics for additional research.

Low BMD and Fractures in Children and Adolescents

Fractures are common in children, and more likely to occur in boys than girls, perhaps because of the greater risk-taking behavior of boys. In a report from Sweden, 42% of boys and 27% of girls experienced a fracture before the age of 17 years.[6] These fractures were usually traumatic, with 24% caused by playing activities, 21% by sports injuries, and 12% by traffic accidents. The most common fracture site was the distal forearm, followed by the phalanges and carpal-metacarpal region. Children with a fracture were at increased risk of having another fracture later in childhood. In a larger population-based cohort study from the United Kingdom, fractures were found to account for 25% of accidents and injuries in childhood.[7] The peak annual incidence rate of fractures was 3% for boys (at age 14 years) and 1.5% for girls (at age 11 years). This rate of fractures is only exceeded in women by age 85 years and never in men.

There is a correlation between bone density and fracture risk in children. A systematic review and meta-analysis of eight case-control studies examined the relationship between measurement of skeletal parameters with a variety of devices (DXA, quantitative computed tomography [QCT], and quantitative ultrasound [QUS]).[8] The findings suggested an increase in fracture risk with lower bone density values. The association of bone density and fracture risk was confirmed in the first prospective study of bone mass and fractures in children, using DXA to measure total body less head (TBLH) areal BMD (aBMD), bone area, and bone mineral content (BMC).[9] In this study of 6,213 children (mean age 9.9 years) followed for 24 months, there was an 89% increased risk of fracture for each standard deviation (SD) decrease in TBLH BMC adjusted for bone area, height, and weight. An association was also reported between fracture risk and low estimated volumetric BMD (vBMD) in a subregion analysis of the humerus. Bone size per se was not related to fracture risk, although children who fractured tended to have a smaller skeleton relative to overall body size. The correlation between estimated humerus vBMD and fracture risk was present regardless of whether the fracture was caused by slight trauma (e.g., falling to ground from a standing position, playground scuffles, low-energy sports injuries), moderate/severe trauma, or severe trauma/severe trauma (e.g., falling downstairs or from a bicycle being moderate trauma and falling from a height more than 3 meters or traffic accident being severe trauma).[10]

Assessment of Skeletal Health in Children and Adolescents

The ISCD states that DXA measurement of the posterior-anterior (PA) spine and TBLH BMC and areal BMD should be part of a comprehensive skeletal health assessment in children and adolescents at high risk for fracture.[2] The hip is not a reliable skeletal site for measurement in growing children because of variability in skeletal development and poor reproducibility (precisions). PA spine and TBLH are recommended because of good accuracy and precision in young patients. In children with linear growth or maturational delay, spine and TBLH BMC and areal BMD results should be adjusted for absolute height or height age, or compared with pediatric reference data that provide age-, gender-, and height-specific Z-scores. An appropriate reference population for calculation of Z-scores must include a sample of the healthy population large enough to characterize the normal variability in bone measures according to gender, age, and race/ethnicity.

DXA should be considered in children and adolescents at the time of clinical presentation of primary bone diseases or potential secondary bone diseases (e.g., chronic inflammatory diseases, endocrine disorders, childhood cancer, or prior nonrenal transplantation). In patients with thalassemia major, these DXA measurements should be done following the first fracture or at age 10 years, whichever is earlier. In children with chronic immobilization, the measurements should be done at fracture presentation. DXA should not be attempted when contractures prevent safe and appropriate positioning of the child.

Soft tissue measurements with whole-body DXA scans may be helpful in evaluating patients with chronic conditions associated with malnutrition (e.g., anorexia nervosa, inflammatory bowel disease, cystic fibrosis) or both muscle and skeletal deficits (e.g., idiopathic juvenile osteoporosis).

Diagnosis of Osteoporosis in Children and Adolescents

The ISCD Official Positions state that the diagnosis of osteoporosis in children and adolescents should *not* be made on the basis of densitometric criteria alone. The diagnosis of osteoporosis requires the presence of both a clinically significant fracture history and low BMC or BMD.[2] A clinically significant fracture is defined by the ISCD as one or more of the following: long bone fracture of the lower extremities, vertebral compression fracture, or two or more long-bone fractures of the upper extremities. Low BMC or areal BMD is defined as a Z-score that is less than or equal to −2.0, adjusted for age, gender, and body size, as appropriate.

Treatment of Osteoporosis in Children and Adolescents

Treatment options for children with osteoporosis are limited because of a paucity of data on efficacy and safety.[4] Few randomized placebo-controlled studies have been conducted in children with skeletal fragility. The fundamental approach to management consists of assuring a healthy lifestyle and adequate nutrition, considering the limitations of the underlying disease state. Physical activity should be encouraged with appropriate measures to minimize the risk of falls. Assistive devices and orthopedic supports should be used when needed. The Institute of Medicine "recommended dietary allowance" (RDA) for calcium and vitamin D are shown in Chapter 6. Adequacy of vitamin D replacement can be assessed by measurement of the serum 25-hydroxy-vitamin D, with a target level of at least 20 ng/mL, with a range of 30 to 50 ng/mL, as suggested in adults, perhaps preferable.[11] Adequate intake of protein and other essential nutrients should be assured, and care should be taken to follow appropriate dietary restrictions, such as a gluten-free diet in children with celiac disease. Effective control of the underlying disease, when possible, is essential. In children with growth retardation, delayed puberty, or hypogonadism, hormonal replacement therapy may be beneficial. Exposure to medications known to have adverse skeletal effects (e.g., glucocorticoids, anticonvulsants) should be minimized, when possible.

None of the drugs used for the treatment of osteoporosis in adults are approved for pediatric patients. However, off-label use of pharmacologic agents may be considered for pediatric patients with osteoporosis who continue to fracture despite all efforts to manage with general measures. Bisphosphonates, the most widely prescribed type of drug for the treatment of osteoporosis in adults, have been studied in children, primarily for those with osteogenesis imperfecta, but also for glucocorticoid-induced osteoporosis, cerebral palsy, muscular dystrophy, burns, idiopathic juvenile osteoporosis, and other pediatric disorders associated with skeletal fragility.[12] A systematic Cochrane review evaluated the efficacy and safety of bisphosphonates (alendronate, clodronate, pamidronate) in six randomized controlled trials, two controlled clinical trials, and one prospective cohort study in children and adolescents with secondary osteoporosis.[13] Although heterogeneity of the studies precluded a combined analysis of the data, it was concluded that further study of bisphosphonates in children with secondary osteoporosis was justified.

The best evidence supporting the use of bisphosphonates in the pediatric population is arguably with osteogenesis imperfecta. A Cochrane systematic review evaluated the efficacy and safety of bisphosphonates in increasing BMD, reducing fracture, and improving clinical function in patients with osteogenesis imperfecta.[14] Eight studies with 403 participants were included. The evidence suggested that oral or intravenous bisphosphonates increased BMD in children and adults with osteogenesis imperfecta, although it was unclear whether fractures were prevented or clinical status was improved.[15]

The long-term effects of bisphosphonates on skeletal growth and fetal skeletal development for pediatric patients who become pregnant as adults are unknown. Although many questions remain regarding the use of bisphosphonates in children, cyclic intravenous pamidronate has become the most common medical therapy for the treatment of children with moderate/severe osteogenesis imperfecta, and is the standard of care at many facilities that treat this disorder.[16]

Selected causes of low bone mass in children and adolescents

Primary bone diseases
- Idiopathic juvenile osteoporosis
- Osteogenesis imperfecta

Inflammatory diseases
- Inflammatory bowel disease
- Juvenile idiopathic arthritis

Chronic immobilization
- Cerebral palsy
- Myopathic disease

Endocrine disorders
- Anorexia nervosa
- Turner syndrome

Hematological diseases
- Thalassemia major
- Acute lymphocytic leukemia

Medications
- Long-term glucocorticoids
- Long-term anticonvulsant therapy

Figure 15.1 Select Diseases of Childhood Associated with High Risk of Fracture.

Adapted from Bishop N, Braillon P, Burnham J, et al. Dual-energy X-ray absorptiometry assessment in children and adolescents with diseases that may affect the skeleton: the 2007 ISCD Pediatric Official Positions. J Clin Densitom. 2008;11(1):29–42.

Summary

Children and adolescents with low-trauma fractures, disorders associated with adverse skeletal effects, and taking medications known to be harmful to the skeleton should be considered for skeletal health assessment. The ISCD has established quality standards for the measurement of BMD and BMC by DXA in children and criteria for the diagnosis of osteoporosis in the pediatric population.[16] The management of skeletal health in children at high risk of fracture includes effective management of the underlying disease, healthy lifestyle, good nutrition, and avoidance of skeletal trauma. For some of these patients, pharmacologic therapy appears to improve BMD, although there is no evidence that any drug reduces fracture risk (Fig. 15.1).

References

1. Klibanski A, Adams-Campbell L, Bassford T, et al. Osteoporosis prevention, diagnosis, and therapy. JAMA. 2001;285(6):785–95.

2. Baim S, Leonard MB, Bianchi ML, et al. Official Positions of the International Society for Clinical Densitometry and executive summary of the 2007 ISCD Pediatric Position Development Conference. J Clin Densitom. 2008;11(1):6–21.

3. WHO Study Group on Assessment of Fracture Risk and its Application to Screening for Postmenopausal Osteoporosis (1994). Assessment of fracture risk and its application to screening for postmenopausal osteoporosis. Geneva: World Health Organization.

4. Bianchi ML. Osteoporosis in children and adolescents. Bone. 2007;41(4):486–95.

5. Rauch F, Plotkin H, DiMeglio L, et al. Fracture prediction and the definition of osteoporosis in children and adolescents: the ISCD 2007 Pediatric Official Positions. J Clin Densitom. 2008;11(1):22–28.

6. Landin LA. Fracture patterns in children. Analysis of 8,682 fractures with special reference to incidence, etiology and secular changes in a Swedish urban population 1950–1979. Acta Orthop Scand Suppl. 1983;202:1–109.

7. Cooper C, Dennison EM, Leufkens HG, et al. Epidemiology of childhood fractures in Britain: a study using the general practice research database. J Bone Miner Res. 2004;19(12):1976–81.

8. Clark EM, Tobias JH, Ness AR. Association between bone density and fractures in children: a systematic review and meta-analysis. Pediatrics. 2006;117(2):e291–97.

9. Clark EM, Ness AR, Bishop NJ, et al. Association between bone mass and fractures in children: a prospective cohort study. J Bone Miner Res. 2006; 21(9): 1489–95.

10. Clark EM, Ness AR, Tobias JH. Bone fragility contributes to the risk of fracture in children, even after moderate and severe trauma. J Bone Miner Res. 2008;23(2):173–79.

11. Binkley N, Lewiecki EM. Vitamin D and common sense. J Clin Densitom. 2011 Apr-;14(2):95–99.

12. Bachrach LK, Ward LM. Clinical review 1: Bisphosphonate use in childhood osteoporosis. J Clin Endocrinol Metab. 2009;94(2):400–09.

13. Ward L, Tricco AC, Phuong P, et al. Bisphosphonate therapy for children and adolescents with secondary osteoporosis. Cochrane Database Syst Rev. 2007;(4):CD005324.

14. Phillipi CA, Remmington T, Steiner RD. Bisphosphonate therapy for osteogenesis imperfecta. Cochrane Database Syst Rev. 2008;(4):CD005088.

15. Cheung MS, Glorieux FH. Osteogenesis Imperfecta: update on presentation and management. Rev Endocr Metab Disord. 2008;9(2):153–60.

16. Bishop N, Braillon P, Burnham J, et al. Dual-energy X-ray aborptiometry assessment in children and adolescents with diseases that may affect the skeleton: the 2007 ISCD Pediatric Official Positions. J Clin Densitom. 2008;11(1):29–42.

Chapter 16

Atypical Femoral Shaft Fractures

Subtrochanteric/femoral shaft fractures (FSF) occurring between the lesser trochanter and the supracondylar flare are not a new entity and represent about 10% of all femoral fractures.[1] They have a bimodal age distribution with peaks among younger and older patients.[2] About 75% are caused by severe trauma, and the remainder occur spontaneously or as a result of low-trauma, mostly in patients with osteoporosis.[1] They are more common in women than men and have a poor prognosis: 14% and 24% mortality in the first 12 and 24 months post fracture, about half the patients do not resume prefracture functionality, and about 71% need alternative accommodation.[3]

Characteristic Features of Atypical FSF

The term *atypical FSF* or atypical femur fracture was coined to differentiate fractures associated with bisphosphonate therapy from "typical" fractures occurring as a result of trauma or the underlying osteoporosis condition (Fig. 16.1).[4]

Basic Science Considerations

Bone turnover maintains a healthy skeleton (see Chapter 2). If bone resorption is inhibited to such an extent that bone under mechanical stress is not replaced by healthier bone, microdamage may occur, accumulate, and lead to insufficiency/stress fractures (IF) (Figs. 16.2, 16.3 and 16.4).[5]

Major Features	Minor Features
Between lesser trochanter and supracondylar flare	Localized periosteal reaction
Minimal or no trauma	Increased cortical thickness of diaphysis
Transverse or short oblique configuration	Prodromal pain in groin or thigh
Noncomminuted	Bilateral fractures
Complete or incomplete	Comorbid conditions and medications

Figure 16.1 Major and Minor Features of Atypical Femoral Shaft Fractures. All Major Features are Required to Meet the Case Definition.

Adapted from Shane E, Burr D, Ebeling PR, et al. Atypical subtrochanteric and diaphyseal femoral fractures: report of a task force of the American Society for Bone and Mineral Research. J Bone Miner Res. 2010;25(11):2267–94, John Wiley & Sons, Inc.

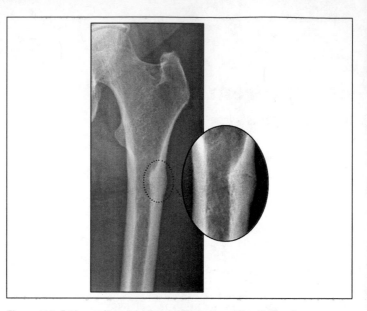

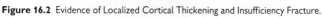

Figure 16.2 Evidence of Localized Cortical Thickening and Insufficiency Fracture.

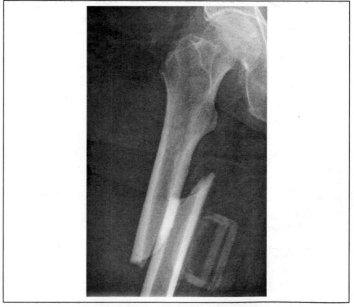

Figure 16.3 Complete Atypical Femoral Shaft Fracture.

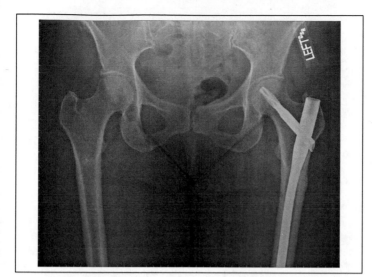

Figure 16.4 Atypical Fragility Fracture After Surgical Repair.

Unlike complete fractures, which heal by endochondral and intramembranous ossification, IF heal by bone remodeling. Theoretically, bisphosphonates may increase the risk of atypical femoral shaft fractures by interfering with the healing process of IF, which may extend and result in complete "atypical" FSF. Atypical FSFs have also been reported in patients treated with non-bisphosphonate compounds (e.g., denosumab) and in some patients never treated for osteoporosis.

Clinical Data

Bisphosphonates have been available for the treatment of osteoporosis in the United States since 1995. It is estimated that in 2004 in the United States, there were about 57 million prescriptions of bisphosphonates,[6] and worldwide there were more than 225 million prescriptions for bisphosphonates by 2007.[7] The number of patients sustaining FSF is so miniscule compared with the total number of prescriptions that a direct causal relationship between bisphosphonates and these fractures cannot be supported. Data from four sources are examined.

Case Studies

Bisphosphonates reduce but do not eliminate the risk of fractures. Therefore, a number of FSF occurring in patients on bisphosphonates could be caused by the underlying osteoporotic process. The two largest reviews of reported cases included 310[4] and 141 cases.[8] After reviewing the available data, the American Society for Bone and Mineral Research (ASMBR) task force concluded that a causal relationship between bisphosphonates and FSF could not be established.[4]

Epidemiologic Studies

In the United States the number of hip fractures decreased from about 600 to 400 per 100,000 patient-years between 1996 (before bisphosphonates) and 2006, whereas the number of FSF has not changed: about 30 per 100,000 patient-years,[9] or has only marginally increased, not proportionally to the decrease in hip fractures.[10] Therefore, it is possible that the decreased incidence of hip fractures is increasing the relative incidence of FSF: from about 30 per 600 in 1996 to 30 per 400 hip fractures per 100,000 patient-years in 2006. If bisphosphonate therapy were associated with an increased risk of FSF, their incidence would have increased inversely proportional to the decrease in hip fractures.

Retrospective Population Studies

The majority of population studies failed to elicit a relationship between bisphosphonate use and FSF. On the contrary, there is evidence of a positive effect of bisphosphonates on FSF and a higher reduction of these fractures in patients highly compliant with bisphosphonate therapy.[11,12]

Prospective Studies

The pivotal prospective, placebo-controlled, double-blind studies (see Chapters 7 and 8) did not document an increase in FSF. Furthermore, a reanalysis of three studies that included some patients on bisphosphonates for 10 years, did not detect increases in FSF in patients on bisphosphonates.[13]

Therefore, the present evidence does not support a direct causative relationship between bisphosphonates and atypical FSF. When these fractures occur in patients on bisphosphonates they may be caused by a low bone turnover rate and therefore do not represent direct adverse effects, but medication overuse or overdose, similar to the hypoglycemia inadvertently induced by administering excessive hypoglycemic agents. Clinicians nevertheless should be alert and recognize patients at risk of developing such fractures, which are different from traumatic or osteoporotic femoral shaft fractures.[14]

Warning Signs

History

Prodromal Symptoms

Many patients on bisphosphonates who sustain FSF report pain in the groin, hip, or thigh weeks to months before sustaining the fracture.[4] In many instances the pain is so severe that patients seek medical help. The pain is often worsened by weight bearing and intensified by standing on one leg.

Comorbidities

Several comorbidities increase the risk of FSF, including rheumatoid arthritis and vitamin D deficiency.[15] Any comorbidity increasing the risk of falls also increases the risk of FSF.

Duration of Bisphosphonate Therapy

Fractures associated with bisphosphonate therapy rarely occur within the first 3 to 5 years of therapy.[13]

Concomitant Medications

Medications leading to bone demineralization and increasing the risk of falls increase the risk of fractures.[16]

Clinical Examination

Tenderness to deep palpation of the femur.

Imaging Studies

A plain x-ray may show evidence of stress or insufficiency fractures. There also may be evidence of localized periosteal reaction on the lateral cortex. Technetium bone scintigraphy reveals localized increased uptake. The sensitivity and specificity of magnetic resonance imaging and computed tomography are better than plain x-rays.

Laboratory Studies

Low levels of markers of bone resorption suggest a low bone turnover rate.

Management

If the patient has symptoms and signs suggestive of a stress or insufficiency fracture and the imaging studies confirm this diagnosis, the antiresorptive medication should be stopped. Causes of secondary osteoporosis, if any, should be identified and managed. Teriparatide[17,18] and prophylactic surgery[19] may be considered.

Conclusion

FSF are much less frequent than hip fractures, and some patients on long-term bisphosphonates may sustain these fractures. The majority are likely to be caused by the underlying osteoporotic condition, rather than bisphosphonate therapy. The present evidence does not support a direct causative relationship between bisphosphonates and FSF. In some rare cases these fractures may result from a low bone turnover rate and an impaired healing process. It may be debated, however, whether this represents a true adverse effect or medication overuse. Notwithstanding, it is recommended to evaluate patients who have been on long-term bisphosphonate therapy (see Chapters 7 and 9). Patients also should be educated about the risk-benefit ratio of bisphosphonates and the early warning signs of atypical FSF.

References

1. Salminen S, Pihlajamäki H, Avikainen V, et al. Specific features associated with femoral shaft fractures caused by low-energy trauma. J Trauma. 1997;43(1):117–22.

2. Singer BR, McLauchlan GJ, Robinson CM, et al. Epidemiology of fractures in 15,000 adults: the influence of age and gender. J Bone Joint Surg Br. 1998;80(2):243–48.

3. Ekström W, Németh G, Samnegard E, et al. Quality of life after a subtrochanteric fracture: a prospective cohort study on 87 elderly patients. Injury. 2009;40(4):371–76.

4. Shane E, Burr D, Ebeling PR, et al. Atypical subtrochanteric and diaphyseal femoral fractures: report of a task force of the American Society for Bone and Mineral Research. J Bone Miner Res. 2010;25(11):2267–94.

5. Mashiba T, Turner CH, Hirano T, et al. Effects of suppressed bone turnover by bisphosphonates on microdamage accumulation and biomechanical properties in clinically relevant skeletal sites in beagles. Bone. 2001;28(5):524–31.

6. Silverman SL, Watts NB, Delmas PD, et al. Effectiveness of bisphosphonates on nonvertebral and hip fractures in the first year of therapy: the risedronate and alendronate (REAL) cohort study. Osteoporos Int. 2007;18(1):25–34.

7. Abughazaleh K, Kawar N. Osteonecrosis of the jaws: what the physician needs to know: practical considerations. Dis Mon. 2011;57(4):231–41.

8. Giusti A, Hamdy NA, Papapoulos SE. Atypical fractures of the femur and bisphosphonate therapy: A systematic review of case/case series studies. Bone. 2010;47(2):169–80.

9. Nieves JW, Bilezikian JP, Lane JM, et al. Fragility fractures of the hip and femur: incidence and patient characteristics. Osteoporos Int. 2010;21(3):399–408.

10. Wang Z, Bhattacharyya T. Trends in incidence of subtrochanteric fragility fractures and bisphosphonate use among the US elderly, 1996–2007. J Bone Miner Res. 2011;26(3):553–60.

11. Abrahamsen B, Eiken P, Eastell R. Subtrochanteric and diaphyseal femur fractures in patients treated with alendronate: a register-based national cohort study. J Bone Miner Res. 2009;24(6):1095–102.

12. Hsiao FY, Huang WF, Chen YM, et al. Hip and subtrochanteric or diaphyseal femoral fractures in alendronate users: a 10-year, nationwide retrospective cohort study in Taiwanese women. Clin Ther. 2011;33(11):1659–67.

13. Black DM, Kelly MP, Genant HK, et al. Bisphosphonates and fractures of the subtrochanteric or diaphyseal femur. N Engl J Med. 2010;362(19):1761–71.

14. Compston J. Pathophysiology of atypical femoral shaft fractures and osteonecrosis of the jaw. Osteoporos Int. 2011;22(12):2951–61.

15. Girgis CM, Sher D, Seibel MJ. Atypical femoral fractures and bisphosphonate use. N Engl J Med. 2010;362(19):1848–49.

16. Ing-Lorenzini K, Desmeules J, Plachta O, et al. Low-energy femoral fractures associated with the long-term use of bisphosphonates: a case series from a Swiss university hospital. Drug Saf. 2009;32(9):775–85.

17. Gomberg SJ, Wustrack RL, Napoli N, et al. Teriparatide, vitamin D, and calcium healed bilateral subtrochanteric stress fractures in a postmenopausal woman with a 13-year history of continuous alendronate therapy. J Clin Endocrinol Metab. 2011;96(6):1627–32.

18. Carvalho NN, Voss LA, Almeida MO, et al. Atypical femoral fractures during prolonged use of bisphosphonates: short-term responses to strontium ranelate and teriparatide. J Clin Endocrinol Metab. 2011;96(9):2675–80.

19. Ha YC, Cho MR, Park KH, et al. Is surgery necessary for femoral insufficiency fractures after long-term bisphosphonate therapy? Clin Orthop Relat Res. 2010;468(12):3393–98.

Chapter 17

Osteonecrosis of the Jaw

Osteonecrosis of the jaw (ONJ) is not a new entity. It may be a serious, difficult to manage, and distressing, but is often mild and asymptomatic. Since its association with bisphosphonates was first reported in 2003,[1] there have been other case reports, case series, and reviews.[2] The terms bisphosphonate-associated osteonecrosis of the jaw (BON) and bisphosphonate-related osteonecrosis of the jaw (BRONJ) were coined to emphasize the association with bisphosphonate therapy. However, ONJ has been reported with denosumab[3,4] and placebo,[5] making the terms BON and BRONJ somewhat obsolete. Another term, antiresorptive agent-induced osteonecrosis of the jaw (ARONJ), has been proposed to designate ONJ associated with any antiresorptive treatment. ONJ is the acronym used here.

ONJ has been defined as the presence of exposed bone in the maxillofacial region for at least 8 weeks after identification by a healthcare provider in a patient who has been exposed to a bisphosphonate and not received radiation therapy to the craniofacial region.[6,7] The mandible is affected more frequently than the maxilla.[8,9]

Incidence

Most patients who develop ONJ have neoplasia, are prescribed much larger doses of bisphosphonates than those for osteoporosis, and are on medications that may predispose to ONJ. In oncology patients, the reported incidence of ONJ varies between 1% and 10% at 3 years.[6,10] Notwithstanding, patients with osteoporosis treated with conventional doses of bisphosphonates or denosumab for osteoporosis have developed ONJ, suggesting that antiresorptive therapy may be a predisposing factor. Its occurrence in patients on placebo, however, illustrates that antiresorptive therapy could be just one of many risk factors

By September 2007 more than 225 million prescriptions for bisphosphonates had been written[11] and in the United States in 2004 there were about 57 million prescriptions for bisphosphonates (see Chapter 16). The risk of ONJ in patients treated with bisphosphonates for osteoporosis is estimated to be between 1 in 10,000 to less than 1 per 100,000 patients,[10,12,13] a risk less than that of injury from motor vehicle accidents.[14]

Factors Predisposing to ONJ

Two main factors increase the risk of ONJ: high dose antiresorptive therapy in oncology patients and invasive dento-alveolar procedures. Other factors include older age, obesity, glucocorticoid intake, alcohol abuse, cigarette smoking, and a number of diseases, including diabetes mellitus, anemia, vitamin D deficiency, pancreatitis, malnutrition, hypothyroidism, hypertension, vascular diseases, renal dialysis, lupus erythematosus, and neoplasia, especially if managed with chemotherapy.[15] Local factors such as tooth extraction, pre-existing periodontal disease, implants, or dentoalveolar surgery increase the risk.[11] ONJ also may occur spontaneously.[15] The present evidence suggests that patients with osteoporosis treated with intravenous bisphosphonates do not have an increased incidence of ONJ during the first 3 years of therapy.[16]

Stages of ONJ

Three stages have been described:[7]

- **Stage 1:** Patient is asymptomatic and often not aware of the condition. Exposed bone has been observed by a health care professional for at least 8 weeks.
- **Stage 2:** Lesion is painful; evidence of superimposed infection: adjacent erythema with or without purulent discharge.
- **Stage 3:** Evidence of extraoral fistulae and/or osteolysis extending to the inferior border and/or pathologic fractures.

    Radiographically, the affected bone may appear mottled with radiolucent and radiodense areas. Bone sequestration may be noted.[7]

These stages were revised in 2009 and Stage 0 was added to include patients with no evidence of exposed necrotic bone, but who have nonspecific symptoms such as pain in the mandible or maxillary sinus, loosening of teeth, and radiographic signs, including alveolar bone loss or resorption not attributable to chronic periodontal disease, changes in trabecular pattern, and inferior alveolar canal narrowing.[17]

Pathophysiology

Various hypotheses have been put forward to explain the sequence of events leading to ONJ.[14,17] The mandible and maxilla are formed by intramembranous as opposed to endochondral ossification, and have a rich blood supply and a high bone turnover rate. They are subjected to frequent repeated mechanical stress, and may come into contact with oral microbacterial flora if the mucosal barrier is breached.[10]

Repeated minor trauma to the jaw bones increases their remodeling activity and vascularity and, therefore, concentration of administered bisphosphonates at these sites. By suppressing bone turnover and angiogenesis, bisphosphonates may lead to microdamage accumulation. Secondary infections set in and further aggravate the problem. This hypothesis, sometimes referred to as the *inside-out hypothesis,* has to be revised in light of ONJ reported in patients on denosumab and placebo. It is also possible that periodontitis or dental procedures damage the mucosa and invite infections from the microbial rich oral flora, which spreads deeper and leads to bone necrosis, the *outside-in hypothesis.*[18]

Management of ONJ

Once a diagnosis of ONJ is made, antiresorptive medication is usually stopped, although there is no evidence that stopping therapy has a beneficial effect on ONJ resolution. There are anecdotal reports that administration of teriparatide may be helpful.[20–22]

- **Stage 1:** Oral antimicrobial (0.12% chlorhexidine) mouth rinses. Scrupulous dental hygiene.
- **Stage 2:** As in stage 1, and: systemic antibiotics, possibly on a long-term basis. Most isolated microbes are sensitive to penicillin. Quinolones, metronidazole, clindamycin, doxycycline, and erythromycin are recommended for patients allergic to penicillin. Microbial culture and sensitivity may be required. Analgesics if required. Superficial debridement.
- **Stage 3:** As in stage 2, and: resection of affected area with immediate or delayed reconstruction.[23] Hyperbaric oxygen and medical ozone may be useful.[24]

Reducing the Risk of ONJ

- Patients should be informed about the risk-benefit ratio of the prescribed medication.
- The patient's gums should be examined—with special attention to dentures—looking for areas of mucosal trauma. This could be done by the treating clinician, and not necessarily a dentist.
- Patients should be instructed about the importance of maintaining good dental hygiene.
- Patients should be educated about ONJ and encouraged to report pain, swelling, exposed bone, or discharge as soon as noticed.
- If possible, anticipated dental interventions, including teeth extractions, should be performed and allowed to heal before the administration of bisphosphonates or denosumab.[16]
- If the patient on bisphosphonates or denosumab needs an invasive dental intervention, it should be done with minimal trauma by a dental specialist with expertise in this area.

References

1. Marx RE. Pamidronate (Aredia) and zoledronate (Zometa) induced avascular necrosis of the jaws: a growing epidemic. J Oral Maxillofac Surg. 2003;61(9):1115–17.

2. Marx RE, Sawatari Y, Fortin M, et al. Bisphosphonate-induced exposed bone (osteonecrosis/osteopetrosis) of the jaws: risk factors, recognition, prevention, and treatment. J Oral Maxillofac Surg. 2005;63(11):1567–75.

3. Akhtar NH, Afzal MZ, Ahmed AA. Osteonecrosis of jaw with the use of denosumab. J Cancer Res Ther. 2011;7(4):499–500.

4. Aghaloo TL, Felsenfeld AL, Tetradis S. Osteonecrosis of the jaw in a patient on Denosumab. J Oral Maxillofac Surg. 2010;68(5):959–63.

5. Grbic JT, Landesberg R, Lin SQ, et al. Incidence of osteonecrosis of the jaw in women with postmenopausal osteoporosis in the health outcomes and reduced incidence with zoledronic acid once yearly pivotal fracture trial. J Am Dent Assoc. 2008;139(1):32–40.

6. Khosla S, Burr D, Cauley J, et al. Bisphosphonate-associated osteonecrosis of the jaw: report of a task force of the American Society for Bone and Mineral Research. J Bone Miner Res. 2007;22(10):1479–91.

7. Advisory Task Force on Bisphosphonate-Related Ostenonecrosis of the Jaws, American Association of Oral and Maxillofacial Surgeons. American Association of Oral and Maxillofacial Surgeons position paper on bisphosphonate-related osteonecrosis of the jaws. J Oral Maxillofac Surg. 2007;65(3):369–76.

8. Woo SB, Hellstein JW, Kalmar JR. Systematic review: bisphosphonates and osteonecrosis of the jaws. Ann Inter Med 2006;144(10):753–761.

9. Otto S, Schreyer C, Hafner S, et al. Bisphosphonate-related osteonecrosis of the jaws - Characteristics, risk factors, clinical features, localization and impact on oncological treatment. J Craniomaxillofac Surg. 2011 Jun 13. [Epub ahead of print]

10. Compston J. Pathophysiology of atypical femoral fractures and osteonecrosis of the jaw. Osteoporos Int. 2011;22(12):2951–61.

11. Abughazaleh K, Kawar N. Osteonecrosis of the jaws: what the physician needs to know: practical considerations. Dis Mon. 2011;57(4):231–41.

12. American Dental Association Council on Scientific Affairs. Dental management of patients receiving oral bisphosphonate therapy: expert panel recommendations. J Am Dent Assoc. 2006;137(8):1144–50.

13. Barasch A, Cunha-Cruz J, Curro FA, et al. Risk factors for osteonecrosis of the jaws: a case-control study from the CONDOR dental PBRN. J Dent Res. 2011;90(4):439–44.

14. Pendrys DG, Silverman SL. Osteonecrosis of the jaws and bisphosphonates. Curr Osteoporos Rep. 2008;6(1):31–38.

15. Shannon J, Shannon J, Modelevsky S, et al. Bisphosphonates and osteonecrosis of the jaw. J Am Geriatr Soc. 2011;59(12):2350–55.

16. Baillargeon J, Kuo YF, Lin YL, et al. Osteonecrosis of the jaw in older osteoporosis patients treated with intravenous bisphosphonates. Ann Pharmacother. 2011;45(10):1199–206.

17. Ruggiero SL, Dodson TB, Assael LA, et al. American Association of Oral and Maxillofacial Surgeons position paper on bisphosphonate-related osteonecrosis of the jaws—2009 update. J Oral Maxillofac Surg. 2009;67(5 Suppl):2–12.

18. Silverman SL, Landesberg R. Osteonecrosis of the jaw and the role of bisphosphonates: a critical review. Am J Med. 2009;122(2 Suppl):S33–45.

19. Marx RE, Cillo JE Jr, Ulloa JJ. Oral bisphosphonate-induced osteonecrosis: risk factors, prediction of risk using serum CTX testing, prevention, and treatment. J Oral Maxillofac Surg. 2007;65(12):2397–410.

20. Lee JJ, Cheng SJ, Jeng JH, et al. Successful treatment of advanced bisphosphonate-related osteonecrosis of the mandible with adjunctive teriparatide therapy. Head Neck. 2011;33(9):1366–71.

21. Chtioui H, Lamine F, Daghfous R. Teriparatide therapy for osteonecrosis of the jaw. N Engl J Med. 2011;364(11):1081–82.

22. Kwon YD, Lee DW, Choi BJ, et al. Short-term teriparatide therapy as an adjunctive modality for bisphosphonate-related osteonecrosis of the jaws. Osteoporos Int. 2012 Jan 5. [Epub ahead of print].

23. Wutzl A, Pohl S, Sulzbacher I, et al. Factors influencing surgical treatment of bisphosphonate-related osteonecrosis of the jaws. Head Neck. 2012;34(2):194–200.

24. Ripamonti CI, Cislaghi E, Mariani L, et al. Efficacy and safety of medical ozone (O(3)) delivered in oil suspension applications for the treatment of osteonecrosis of the jaw in patients with bone metastases treated with bisphosphonates: Preliminary results of a phase I-II study. Oral Oncol. 2011;47(3):185–90.

Index

Page numbers followed by t indicate a table. Italicized page numbers indicate a figure or photo